These Three Things

Lisa Jenkins • Terri Averi • Tina Opina

These Three Things

A Guide for Navigating the Dementia Journey

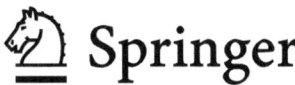
Springer

Lisa Jenkins
Supportive Care
Community LIFE
Pittsburgh, PA, USA

Terri Averi
Supportive Care
Community LIFE
Munhall, PA, USA

Tina Opina
Supportive Care
Community LIFE
New Kensington, PA, USA

ISBN 978-3-031-69393-9   ISBN 978-3-031-69394-6   (eBook)
https://doi.org/10.1007/978-3-031-69394-6

This Springer imprint is published by the registered company Springer Nature Switzerland AG
The registered company address is: Gewerbestrasse 11, 6330 Cham, Switzerland

If disposing of this product, please recycle the paper.

Foreword

In the pages that follow, you will embark on a journey of understanding and empowerment. This book, a ray of hope amidst the often-challenging landscape of dementia, offers an insightful collection of caregiver tips that are not just practical but also nurturing. Dementia touches countless lives rippling through families and communities leaving a trail of questions and uncertainties in its wake, yet within the heart of this experience lies an opportunity for growth, connection, and the discovery of strength within oneself. As you delve into these pages, you'll discover invaluable insights on how to navigate the complexities of dementia with grace and resilience. Whether you're a caregiver, a family member, or even someone grappling with dementia themselves, these tips provide a lifeline of support. Drawing upon a wealth of knowledge, experience, and empathy, Terri, Tina, and Lisa offer straightforward solutions that allow a caregiver to find solace even in the face of challenge. It reminds us that, amidst the trials of caring for someone with dementia, we should focus on "these three things".... moments of joy, connection, and shared experiences that can enrich our lives in unexpected ways. May these pages serve as a guiding light forward toward demystifying the complexities of dementia, allowing more space for compassion and joy. Embrace this journey, for within it lies the potential to create meaningful moments and discover the power of caregiving with unwavering love.

With deepest regards,

AVP Medical Services SNP   Kalpana Char
UPMC Health Plan
Cheswick, PA, USA

These Three Things

Activities of Daily Living (ADLs)
- Refusing to brush their teeth
- Afraid to take a shower
- Refusing to take a shower
- Providing nail care
- Disrobing
- Getting dressed
- Not changing clothes
- Not dressing appropriately for the weather
- Refusing to put on their coat
- Maintaining independence

Behaviors
- Communication struggles
- Repeating stories or questions
- Calling you repeatedly
- Arguing
- Hoarding (non-food)
- Preventing aggressive behavior
- Managing aggression
- Difficult behaviors in public
- Public sexual behaviors
- Inappropriate touching of others
- Inappropriate language
- Anxiety/fear
- Being afraid
- Hallucinations
- Delusions
- Paranoia
- Shadowing
- Making false accusations

- Continuous pacing
- Sundowning
- A full moon
- Spitting
- Hyperorality (hyper oral)
- Picking or scratching at skin
- Not wanting to get in the car
- Not wanting to get out of the car
- Taking something that is not theirs
- Thinking that something belongs to them that is not theirs

Caregiving
- Accepting that your loved one has this disease
- Not recognizing you
- Feeling guilty about taking time for yourself
- Feeling like I'm going to lose it
- Managing the long-term stress of caregiving
- You being sick
- Needing to be away from the person
- Explaining dementia to young children
- Family members not agreeing on care
- Needing help from others
- Looking for community resources

Change
- Change
- Change of seasons
- Daylight savings time
- Moving to a new living environment
- Transitioning from one activity to the next
- Leaving a room to go to another
- A loved one passing away

Medical
- Being asked "What is wrong with me?"
- Their sadness or depression
- Not wanting to take medication
- The person being sick
- A urinary tract infection
- Suspecting they are in pain, but they can't communicate it
- Going to appointments
- A dentist appointment
- A podiatry appointment
- Keeping them hydrated
- Initiating eating

- Forgetting that they've eaten
- Hoarding food
- Pocketing food

Safety
- Elopement risk
- An elopement
- Smoking that has become unsafe
- Smoking in an inappropriate/non-smoking environment
- Unsafe cooking
- Driving that has become worrisome
- Falls
- Using ambulatory assistance devices
- Mismanaging finances
- Safe proofing the home from chemicals
- Repeatedly calling 911
- Struggling to care for a pet
- Unnecessarily adjusting the thermostat

Sleep
- Wanting to go to bed too early
- Not sleeping through the night
- Having their days and nights mixed up
- Keeping them safe while you're asleep

Socializing
- Going to the hairdresser
- Attending a special event
- Holiday celebrations
- Having visitors
- Visiting in a facility
- Not having a meaningful visit
- Leaving the facility after a visit

Toileting
- Being unable to verbalize the need to go to the bathroom
- Not wanting to use the bathroom
- Not accepting assistance with changing incontinence products
- Urinating in the house
- Public urination

Prologue: These Three Things

As you care for a person with dementia, there are many changes and situations you will be faced with handling. The purpose of *These Three Things* is to provide you with three concrete options of things to try when each situation occurs. Three things to remember:

1. There is no way that we can cover every single situation that may arise. Dementia is unpredictable. This book contains 99 scenarios; however, we have left room at the end for you to document situations that you experience.
2. Not every suggestion is going to work for every situation. Everyone travels the journey differently. What does not work today, may work tomorrow. What does work today, may not work tomorrow. Therefore, our hope is that our tips and techniques will help you to think critically and creatively as you problem solve your specific situations.
3. We often focus our energy on the person with dementia; you must remember that you play a significant role in this journey, too. You will find information in this book about ways that you can care for yourself as well.

We know that caring for a person with dementia takes a lot of time and energy. Our goal is to make this book quick and easy to use. We share information about dementia, caregiver stress and brain health. The majority of the book focuses on *These Three Things* and is divided into the following categories:

Activities of Daily Living (ADLs), Behaviors, Caregiving, Change, Medical, Nutrition, Safety, Sleep, Socializing, Toileting

Each category is broken down into specific scenarios. For example, if the person you are caring for is not wanting to brush their teeth, you will look that up in the index, go to page 53 and find the following:

When faced with the challenge of *refusing to brush their teeth*, try *These Three Things…*

1. Use mirror image—brush your teeth, too.
2. Put on music and brush to the beat.
3. Make sure the toothpaste is not too minty.
    They may not be able to communicate that the toothpaste is burning their mouth.

Pick one of the suggestions to try. You do not have to use these approaches in order. Use what feels right to you.

If that one works, great! If it doesn't work the first time, we encourage you to try the same technique three times. If after the third time you still haven't had success, move on to try a different approach.

You are not alone on this journey. We have seen all of these approaches in action. Our hope is that you find success or inspiration that makes your important job as a caregiver a little bit easier. Take a deep breath and try *These Three Things*.

Contents

Chapter 1
What Is Dementia?

Once You've Seen One Person with Dementia, You've Seen One Person with Dementia

We are all individuals. No two people are alike. Just as your life journey is your own, your experience with dementia will be your own. There are many similarities between the various forms of dementia, but also great differences. Therefore, as we dive into defining what is dementia, we will talk very broadly.

Dementia
A general term for loss of memory, language, problem-solving, and other thinking abilities that are severe enough to interfere with daily life. It is not a specific disease [1].

Dementia is an umbrella term for a clustering of conditions that impacts the brain [2] (Fig. 1.1). Reports vary on the exact number of types of dementias. While there are many types of dementia, the tips and techniques we are going to explore are relative to any type of dementia.

The most prevalent symptom of dementia is memory loss. Additional symptoms [2] that you may see include but are not limited to:

- Difficulty with problem-solving
- Reduced judgment
- Cognitive changes
- Sensory changes
- Difficulty with communication
- Reduced ability to plan, organize, or reason
- Difficulty handling complex tasks

© The Author(s), under exclusive license to Springer Nature Switzerland AG 2024
L. Jenkins et al., *These Three Things*,
https://doi.org/10.1007/978-3-031-69394-6_1

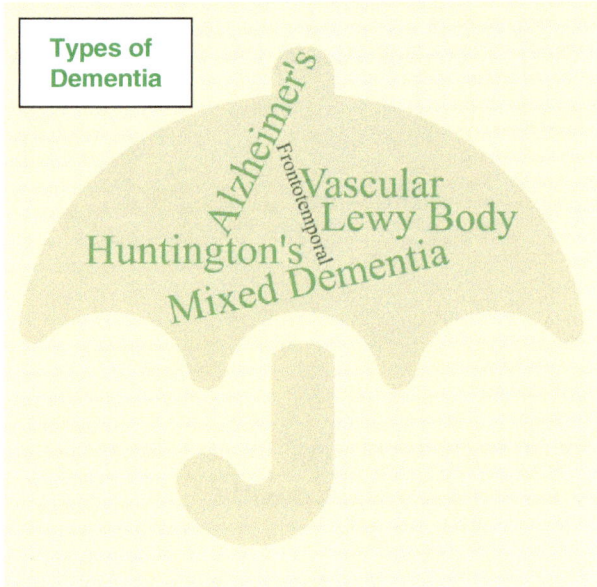

Fig. 1.1 The dementia umbrella

- Change in motor function
- Psychological changes
- Changes in personality and behaviors
- Mood swings
- Agitation
- Social withdrawal

Dementia is a progressive disease. Even though not everyone will experience all of the above-mentioned symptoms at the same time or to the same intensity, the common denominator is that any combination of these symptoms will impact the quality of life [3].

Dementia causes damage to the brain and brain cells. The damage interferes with the ability of the brain cells to communicate with each other. When brain cells cannot communicate efficiently, thinking, behavior, and feelings can be affected. Depending on what part of the brain is impacted will determine what symptoms you will see.

Look at the image of the three brains below. Figure 1.2 The brain on the left is a healthy brain. The two brains on the right illustrate a diseased brain. Please note that all dementias will result in the shrinkage of the brain [4]. In the impacted brain, you can see that shrinking will create gaps which result in the loss of connective paths for information to travel [5]. Think of the pipes under your sink. They are all connected allowing the water to flow freely and with direction. If you removed a pipe or a pipe became clogged, the water would spill out or have nowhere to go becoming problematic. Depending on where the pipe is located will depend on what area of your house is impacted. Your kitchen sink? The shower? The laundry room? As

Progression of Alzheimer's Disease

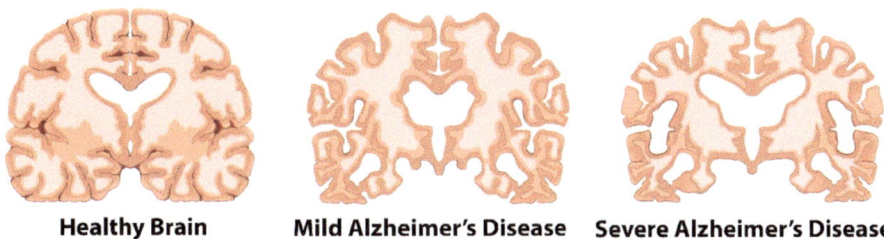

Healthy Brain   **Mild Alzheimer's Disease**   **Severe Alzheimer's Disease**

Fig. 1.2 Healthy brain vs. brains with Alzheimer's disease [4]

different areas of the brain are impacted, different symptoms or behaviors will be present. For example, areas that affect reasoning, sensory, communication, or memory.

The progression of dementia depends on a variety of factors. There may be times that you might notice a sequence of small changes over a period of time. Other times the progression may plateau for a month or even a year. Sometimes the progression will happen quickly. Something may happen like a medical condition or life change where you see a decline. The rate of progression and life expectancy will be impacted by the specific type of dementia [6].

There is a difference between an acute rapid onset change versus the gradual progression of dementia. A medical condition that can result in an acute change in behavior is delirium. Delirium and dementia have many overlapping symptoms. The main differences are that delirium has a much more rapid onset and it is often reversible [7].

Delirium
Is an abrupt onset of reduced orientation or awareness to the environment in contrast to dementia which is a gradual process leading to disturbance in the core features, and attention is affected much later in the disease course [7].

A diagnosis of dementia may not be clear despite a variety of symptoms being present. Because dementia is unique to each individual, you may not always pick up on the signs and symptoms in its early stages. To be definitively diagnosed, please follow-up with your medical provider.

Dementia has a wide impact. Today, 55 million people have a diagnosis of dementia worldwide. This number will only grow as the population ages. One in three seniors die with a diagnosis of Alzheimer's disease or another form of dementia. The economic impact of dementia is $257 billion/year in the United States [8]. The impact goes far beyond the person with the diagnosis. It is estimated that 65–75% of people with dementia are cared for at home by family members.

Approximately two third of dementia caregivers are women. 34% of dementia caregivers age 65 or older. The impact of dementia spreads to the financial, emotional, and physical health of caregivers [9].

References

1. What is dementia? Alzheimer's Association. https://www.alz.org/alzheimers-dementia/what-is-dementia#diagnosis.
2. What is dementia? Symptoms, types and diagnosis. National Institute of Aging. https://www.nia.nih.gov/health/what-is-dementia#signs.
3. How dementia progresses. Alzheimer's Society. https://www.alzheimers.org.uk/about-dementia/symptoms-and-diagnosis/how-dementia-progresses#:~:text=Dementia%20is%20progressive.,progressing%20in%20%27three%20stages%27.
4. An anatomy of human brain, by brgfx of FreePik. https://www.freepik.com/free-vector/anatomy-human-brain_2413746.htm#fromView=search&page=3&position=4&uuid=bad5de87-58b3-4832-bcdc-c24eb54841e6.
5. Blinkouskaya Y, Weickenmeier J. Brain shape changes associated with cerebral atrophy in healthy aging and Alzheimer's disease. Front Mech Eng. 2021;7:705653. https://doi.org/10.3389/fmech.2021.705653.
6. Dementia life expectancy: progression and stages after diagnosis. Agespace: Taking Care of Care. https://www.agespace.org/dementia/life-expectancy.
7. Gogia B, Fang X. Differentiating delirium versus dementia in the elderly. In: StatPearls. Treasure Island, FL: StatPearls Publishing; 2024. https://www.ncbi.nlm.nih.gov/books/NBK570594/.
8. Alzheimer's Association. 2023 Alzheimer's disease facts and figures. Alzheimers Dement. 2023;19(4):1598–695. https://doi.org/10.1002/alz13016.
9. Profile of older adults with dementia and their caregivers brief. ASPE Office of the Assistant Secretary for Planning and Evaluation; 2019. https://aspe.hhs.gov/reports/profile-older-adults-dementia-their-caregivers-issue-brief-0.

Chapter 2
Dementia and Communication

Communication is defined as the process of understanding and sharing meaning [1].

Communication is verbal and nonverbal. Communication involves a sender and receiver [1]. When one of those people has some type of impairment, verbal and nonverbal communication will be impacted. A person with dementia will have problems with both sending and receiving information. This will influence the process of understanding and being understood. Struggles with communication can be a cause of great frustration for both the caregiver and the person with dementia. The impact on communication will also progress or change over time [2].

With verbal communication, a person with dementia as the sender of information may not be able to think of the word they want, use a word incorrectly, speak in a word salad or have decreased speech. As the disease progresses, they will eventually become nonverbal. With verbal communication, a person with dementia as the receiver of information may have trouble following the story line, take your words literally, not be able to process what you're saying or struggle to follow simple commands [2, 3].

With nonverbal communication, a person with dementia as the sender of information may display facial expressions that do not match their verbal communication or behaviors. They may develop a flat affect or show no emotion at all. With nonverbal communication, the person with dementia as the receiver will be very in tune to your nonverbal cues. They can sense when you are distracted, stressed, angry, or sad. They are unable to accurately process what all of this means. They may also mirror your behavior or emotion [2, 3].

Understanding communication plays a vital role in providing care for the person with dementia. While it can seem complicated and confusing, here are some simple tips that can ease the stress around communicating with the one for which you are caring.

L. Jenkins et al., *These Three Things*, https://doi.org/10.1007/978-3-031-69394-6_2

1. Don't argue. This is an argument you will lose every time. For example:

   (a) If they say it is raining outside when it is in fact sunny, grab that umbrella as you walk out the door. It is now raining in your sunny world.
   (b) If they think that it is 1976 and they need to be home to meet their children from school, don't correct them to the present moment. Instead, use a therapeutic truth saying "It's not time yet." or "We'll leave soon."

2. Use five words or less, speak slowly and focus on one subject at a time. When communicating try not to be too wordy. For example, "Come with me." "It's time to eat." "Can you help me?" "Let's go."

3. Simplify choices. For example, instead of "What do you want to wear today?" ask "Red or blue shirt?" while showing them the two shirts.

4. Avoid open-ended questions. For example, knowing that her sister Sally stopped by the house, ask "Was today good?" instead of "What did you do today?"

5. Limit distractions—Be aware of what is happening around you. Is the TV too loud? Are there multiple conversations happening in the room? Is the window open magnifying the sounds of birds or passing cars?

6. Make sure you are in front of them at eye level if possible, while speaking slowly. If they are seated, kneel in front of them or pull up a chair. If you are off to the side, try to be on their dominant side. Standing over them can be intimidating. Avoid yelling from a different room or from behind them.

7. Be aware of your reactions both verbal and nonverbal. For example

   (a) People with dementia often lose their filter. They may vocalize their thoughts without holding back. "That shirt looks really ugly on you." "You are getting chubby." Rather than acting shocked or firing back, simply roll with it. Don't take their words personally.
   (b) If something shocking or unexpected happens or is said, try not to react with a big gasp or shocked face. For example, they may start to swear when they have rarely sworn before.

8. Be an investigator—Look beyond the words. What is the meaning behind what they are trying to say? For example, if they say they want to go home, but they are home. They may be looking to find comfort, security, activity, or a hug.

9. Use written notes or pictures if they are unable to understand spoken words. For example, place a picture of a toilet on the bathroom door or a stop sign on the back of the front door to prevent them from leaving.

10. Use spaced retrieval. This assists with recalling information by providing it to them in written format and then referring to it. For example, if the person is repeatedly asking for their car and their car is no longer at their home do the following:

    (a) Write on a piece of paper or index card: "Your car is at mechanics."
    (b) Place it somewhere where they will see it often—on the refrigerator, on the end table next to their recliner or on the bathroom mirror.

(c) When they ask the question, answer it without correcting them and refer to the note.
(d) After a while, gently refer to the note.
(e) Research has shown that some people will eventually stop asking the question knowing to look at the note without the reminder [4, 5].

Overall, be a compassionate listener. We are constantly in communication with each other whether it is verbal or nonverbal. There are going to be times of great frustration as you and the person with dementia find your way through the changes that will occur. For them, there will be no control over what is happening to them. Hold tight to compassion.

References

1. Business communication for success. University of Minnesota; 2015. https://open.lib.umn.edu/businesscommunication/chapter/1-2-what-is-communication/.
2. Banovic S, Zunic LJ, Sinanovic O. Communication difficulties as a result of dementia. Mater Sociomed. 2018;30(3):221–4. https://doi.org/10.5455/msm.2018.30.221-224.
3. Alzheimer's disease: how the disease progresses. Mayo Clinic. https://www.mayoclinic.org/diseases-conditions/alzheimers-disease/in-depth/alzheimers-stages/art-20048448.
4. Creighton AS, van der Ploeg ES, O'Connor DW. A literature review of spaced-retrieval interventions: a direct memory intervention for people with dementia. Int Psychogeriatr. 2013;25(11):1743–63. https://doi.org/10.1017/S1041610213001233.
5. Malone M. The spaced retrieval technique: a how-to for SLPs. SpeechPathology.com. 2022. p. 20503. www.speechpathology.com.

Chapter 3
Dementia and Sensory Changes

Sensory changes occur with normal aging. When senses are impaired, it will impact the ability to process information. Adding a diagnosis of dementia will heighten the impact, which in turn will influence how we provide care. People with dementia may not be aware of the changes in their senses. Look at how the changes in senses effect both the person with dementia and how you care for them [1, 2].

With age, the sense of smell is often the first to change. One consequence of this loss is increased safety risk. For example, they may not be able to smell gas or smoke from a fire or spoiled food. This can raise concerns about their safety if they live alone. A person's day-to-day living may also be effected. A diminished sense of smell can change their desire to eat. Body hygiene can be impacted as the person is unable to smell body odor or an episode of incontinence. They may not recognize that they have applied too much perfume or cologne [1–3].

As a caregiver, it will be important to ensure that you have functioning smoke and carbon monoxide detectors. If a person lives alone, you will want to monitor their food to ensure that it is not spoiled. Providing more shelf stable items can reduce the risk of spoilage. Conversations around hygiene may be difficult. You may need to be creative in ways that you encourage bathing, cleanliness, and changing of clothes. There are also items that you can purchase that can help in this area such as adult diaper genies and automatic air fresheners. More specific interventions can be found throughout *These Three Things* (see Chap. 7).

Closely related to smell is the sense of taste. One area of life greatly affected by the loss of taste is eating. When one cannot taste, the desire to eat diminishes. This can lead to changes in weight, energy level, and mood. Sweet taste buds remain the longest leading to cravings for sugary foods. A person may continue to add more and more salt to their food as they can no longer taste a small amount. Lack of taste may cause adverse health concerns as the person is increasing their use of salt and sugar. They may also not taste when food is spoiled which can result in gastrointestinal problems. How a person experiences flavor may change leading one to enjoy

L. Jenkins et al., *These Three Things*,
https://doi.org/10.1007/978-3-031-69394-6_3

flavors they never liked before, disliking something that has been a lifelong favorite or eating food combinations that may seem odd [1, 2].

As a caregiver you need to find your comfort level with the balance of nutrition versus quality of life. Is it more important that their blood sugar remain stable or that they eat the ice cream they love for dinner when they are rejecting the meat and vegetables? That is a question that only you can answer for your situation. You may want to limit saltshakers or replace salt with a salt substitute. You can also add rice to the saltshakers to help control the flow of what comes out and gives the appearance of a full shaker. If this is an area of great concern, ask your medical provider for a referral to a dietitian. Additional interventions can be found throughout *These Three Things* (Chap. 7).

As we age, our vision may change drastically. There will be a change in depth perception resulting in increased risk for falls and misjudging distances [4]. One's visual field will change as the peripheral vision gradually becomes narrower. The process of shifting of one's gaze may become slower. There may also be diminished ability to distinguish movement, colors, and faces. Pupils will take longer to adapt to light [5].

The person may also misinterpret what they see. Crumbs may be misinterpreted as bugs or window decorations misinterpreted as people looking in at them.

As a caregiver, recognizing visual changes and taking simple actions could avert potential problems and safety risks. Be mindful of the lighting in your home. Bright lights will be overstimulating, use of side table lamps may be a better choice. Maintain clear pathways throughout the home. Keep decorations simple. Use contrasting colors for items such as plates, toilet seats, and signs. Approach people from the front as discussed in the chapter on Dementia and Communication. Additional interventions can be found throughout *These Three Things* (Chap. 7).

The sense of touch is affected by aging. People may experience a loss of sensation reducing the ability to feel heat, cold, discomfort, or pain. The person with dementia may not interpret the increased safety risks that come with this loss of sensation. The change in sense of touch may also result in difficulty managing clothing such as buttons and zippers. Touch can help to create a sense of comfort and well-being through a soft blanket or a pet's fur. Losing this sense of touch can increase feelings of isolation and loneliness [4, 5].

As a caregiver, it is important to be aware that changes in touch may present in ways that are not obvious such as too tight shoes and rough clothing tags. Monitor skin for cuts and bruises that may not be apparent to the person. Ensure that the water heater is set at a safe temperature. Additional interventions can be found throughout *These Three Things* (Chap. 7).

Hearing is usually the last sense to remain [6]. Sound has the power to stimulate the brain. Without that power, the risk of cognitive decline and atrophy in the brain is higher. Decreased hearing can alter your perception of what is happening around you and create difficulty in processing background noise. Hearing loss can also create a communication barrier. Following a conversation can be challenging. This can result in lack of social interactions leading to isolation [1, 2].

As a caregiver, recognizing hearing loss is important as it impacts communication. There are multiple devices that can assist with improving hearing such as hearing aides and pocket talkers. Consult with your medical provider for referrals. Be cognizant of multiple sound stimulants at once—the dog barking, the TV on, and a fan blowing while you're trying to have a conversation. Refer to the chapter on Dementia and Communication for more tips on strategies. Recognize that the person may not be hearing all of the words you're saying. Their brain may automatically attempt to fill in the gaps. This can lead to misunderstanding or paranoia. Even when people can't hear us, they can respond to our nonverbal cues. Additional interventions, can be found throughout *These Three Things* (Chap. 7).

While sensory changes occur with normal aging, the impact of those changes will be heightened by the changing brain. As the caregiver, being aware of these changes can help to determine the best course of action when providing care.

References

1. Cavazzana A, Röhrborn A, Garthus-Niegel S, Larsson M, Hummel T, Croy I. Sensory-specific impairment among older people. An investigation using both sensory thresholds and subjective measures across the five senses. PLoS One. 2018;13(8):e0202969. https://doi.org/10.1371/journal.pone.0202969.
2. Take care of your senses: the science behind sensory loss and dementia risk. National Institute on Aging; 2023. https://www.nia.nih.gov/news/take-care-your-senses-science-behind-sensory-loss-and-dementia-risk.
3. How smell and taste change as your age. National Institute on Aging. https://www.nia.nih.gov/health/smell-and-taste.
4. Shuyi O, Zheng C, Lin Z, Zhang X, Li H, Fang Y, Hu Y, Yu H, Wu G. Risk factors of falls in elderly patients with visual impairment. Front Public Health. 2022;10:984199. https://doi.org/10.3389/fpubh.2022.984199. Erratum in: Front Public Health. 2022;10:1087472.
5. Your aging eyes: How you see as times goes by. News in Health; 2011. https://newsinhealth.nih.gov/2011/01/your-aging-eyes.
6. Blundon EG, Gallagher RE, Ward LM. Electrophysiological evidence of preserved hearing at the end of life. Sci Rep. 2020;10(1):10336. https://doi.org/10.1038/s41598-020-67234-9.

Chapter 4
Dementia: Behaviors and Emotions

Behaviors
Behavioral disturbances in dementia are drastic changes in behavior which may seem to occur out of nowhere. They can include changes in behavior, perception, thoughts, and mood [1].

In dementia, behaviors that a person has displayed throughout their lives will most likely remain, may be heightened or new ones may appear. Dealing with the heightened or new behaviors may be a challenge. The most important thing to remember is that your loved one is your loved one even though they are behaving differently. As the caregiver, learning to manage behaviors can help to maintain the relationship. You did not sign up to be a caregiver. The person you are caring for did not sign up to have dementia.

As you read about these behaviors, it is important to keep *These Three Things* in mind:

1. Once you've seen one person with dementia, you've seen one person with dementia.
2. Every person will go through this disease process differently.
3. This is not a comprehensive list.

It would be impossible to capture every scenario that you might experience. This chapter is a general description of the behaviors and possible rationales of why they are occurring. *These Three Things*, Chap. 7, will give you suggestions on how to manage behaviors.

There are a variety of causal factors for a behavior such as a progression of the dementia, environmental, sensory, or a medical condition. If you see a sudden and/ or unexplained onset or change in a behavior, it is important to make your medical

L. Jenkins et al., *These Three Things*, https://doi.org/10.1007/978-3-031-69394-6_4

provider aware. This is important as some of these behaviors can be treated with medical interventions or could mask a delirium.

Let's look at how these behavioral changes impact the person with dementia and the caregiver.

Aggression

Aggression is the forceful or overly assertive pursuit of one's aims and interests [2]. This can be a physical act or one of intimidation. Aggression may look like standing up while yelling, a raised fist, throwing something, posturing, charging toward you or physical contact. Stay alert—the body language may be incongruent. For example, he may be smiling, but when you walk toward him, he raises his fist. Having dementia can be very frustrating. The person you are caring for may not understand what is happening or be able to communicate what they are thinking or feeling. This can lead to aggressive behavior. Aggression can also come out of nowhere.

Anger

Anger is a strong feeling of annoyance, displeasure, or hostility [3]. Like aggression, anger may be a result of frustration. There can be a lot to be angry about—they may not process what is happening. They may not be able to explain what they are feeling. Their lives have been forever changed by this diagnosis. Some people may be easily evoked to anger. People can demonstrate angry behaviors even though the situation doesn't warrant it. The behavior and the situation may not match. Anger can be loud or a quiet stewing. Anger can come across through their body language or through sounds. You as the caregiver may feel anger as well. It is important to keep in mind that the person you are caring for may mirror your emotions. While it can be difficult in the moment, managing your anger can lead to a more positive interaction.

Anxiety

Anxiety is a feeling of worry, nervousness, or unease typically about an imminent event or something with an uncertain outcome [4]. People with dementia live in the moment. They may be unable to remember what just happened or not be able to process what is about to happen next. Some people blissfully live in this world. Others may experience great anxiety. People with dementia may mentally travel back in time. They may be feeling anxious about a situation that happened 50 years ago. The intense emotion of anxiety can be demonstrated in many ways including pacing, crying, questioning, and nervous tremors. This is another situation where you as a caregiver may be experiencing this emotion. It is important to keep in mind that the person you are caring for may mirror you. While it may be difficult in the moment, managing your anxiety will lead to a more positive interaction.

Delusions

A delusion is a false belief or judgment about external reality, held despite incontrovertible evidence to the contrary, occurring especially in mental conditions [5]. Paranoia is a frequent type of delusion. For example, the person with dementia may think that you are an imposter. You're someone impersonating their daughter who has been sent to watch them. They may think that you are having an affair. They may think that you are trying to poison them with the medicine you are giving them. To them, these situations are real. Their perceptions of reality are altered. Delusions can come out of nowhere. Delusions can also be influenced by what a person is watching on TV, reading, or an overhead conversation.

Demanding

"I want what I want when I want it!" Patience can often diminish for a person with dementia. Their world may become very small and their ability to comprehend time may be hampered. They may also not be able to "read" the situation at hand. Even though you are elbow deep in carving the Thanksgiving turkey, they need you to get them Jeanne's phone number right NOW and you have never heard of Jeanne. Demanding can be displayed as loud, forceful, and repetitive. Not addressing the situation can lead to anger and aggression.

Elopement

Elopement is "when a (person) wanders away or leaves an area without supervision or authorization and presents a safety threat to the (person) and/or others" [6]. Six out of ten people with dementia will elope [7] at some point during their dementia journey. It is impossible to predict with 100% certainty when and if an elopement will take place; however, there are several factors that can help you to identify an increased elopement risk. A few examples are:

- Talking about situations from the past such as having to pick the kids up from school or being late for an appointment.
- Exit seeking—going to doors and rattling doorknobs, pacing

- Any change—a new caregiver, moving to a new residence, a different routine
- Boredom

Fear

Fear is an emotion. It can come from many different places.

- Not remembering what just happened.
- Not knowing what is coming next.
- Not recognizing who is in the room with them.
- Not being able to process time or place.

The natural fight-or-flight response to a stressful or frightening situation—whether real or perceived—will determine one's reaction to fear [8]. Identifying that the root cause of a behavior is fear will help you determine how to respond.

Hallucinations

A hallucination is a false perception of objects or events involving your senses: sights, sounds, smell, touch, and taste. They seem real to the person experiencing them, but they are not [9, 10]. Potential medical causes for hallucinations should be ruled out. There are certain types of dementia where hallucinations are more common [11]. Examples of hallucinations include

- Seeing someone looking in their window
- Hearing someone call their name or music playing
- Feeling bugs crawling up their leg

Hoarding

Hoarding is persistent difficulty getting rid of or parting with possessions due to a perceived need to save the item [12]. Some of the more common items that people hoard are food, mail, papers, or clothes. There may be multiple reasons why hoarding behaviors occur.

- It can be due to looking for control in a situation where they have no control.
- Items around them may provide them with a sense of comfort and security when they are feeling isolated.
- A person may experience anxiety surrounding understanding that they might lose something.

- People may have difficulty parting with items due to a perceived need to save them.
- Lifelong collecting can become out of control when dementia reduces your impulse control.

Hyperorality (Hyper Oral)

A person who is hyper oral has an excessive tendency to overeat, eat things that are not food or constantly place things in their mouth. Risks of this behavior include choking, pocketing food, soft tissue damage, dental injuries, and accidental poisoning [13].

Inappropriate Language

People with dementia often lose their filter using words that they would have previously recognized as inappropriate, offensive, or hurtful. For example, someone who rarely swore may use swear words all the time. Racial or ethnic slurs may be spoken. They may tell off-color jokes at the dinner table or not think twice about telling someone they are fat. It is important to not take things personally. It is the disease talking. This is not a conscious behavior. Other times you just need to laugh and let it go.

Inappropriate Sexual Behaviors

Sexuality is a basic need throughout the lifespan. There is a need for touch and comfort. The lack of social awareness that may come with dementia can lead this appropriate behavior into becoming inappropriate. Examples of inappropriate sexual behaviors may include masturbating or disrobing in public, sexual touching of others, or making sexual references.

Picking/Scratching Skin

There are many reasons why a person with dementia may pick or scratch at their skin. They may be doing this in an attempt to self-soothe or when struggling to verbally communicate an emotion, discomfort, or need. It can also be caused by stress and anxiety. They may be unable to control themselves or forget that they aren't supposed to touch that area.

Repetition

A person with dementia may forget that they've already said or done something which can result in repetitive behaviors. This could be calling you repeatedly, asking the same question over and over or doing an action multiple times. These behaviors are typically not harmful to the person with dementia, but may be stressful, annoying, or exhausting for the caregiver.

Restlessness

Restless behavior is when a person is fidgety and has the need to move. They may be pacing, unable to sit still, pulling at their clothes, or wringing their hands. This may be a concern if it goes on for long periods of time. For example, a person who is pacing for hours on end may become tired increasing the risk for falls. Causes of restlessness may include boredom, pain, discomfort, the need to use the bathroom or searching for something.

Shadowing

A person with dementia may struggle with what to do next or become increasingly disoriented. This may evoke fear creating a sense of being unsafe and a need for security. As a result, they may look to those around them for direction which may lead to them literally following a person around going where they go or doing what they're doing. Though not particularly dangerous, shadowing can create a constant sense of stress for the caregiver.

Sleep Disturbance

Sleep is an important part of our health—both for the person with dementia and their caregiver. People with dementia may

- Sleep more during the day (especially as the disease progresses)
- Wake more frequently in the middle of the night and have trouble falling back asleep
- Experience sleep reversal (having their days and nights mixed up) [14].

With an already compromised brain, the growing exhaustion caused by sleep disturbances can have a greater impact on the person with dementia resulting in them needing more support. Being a caregiver in and of itself is exhausting. Providing care will be extra challenging when you are also feeling exhausted.

Stubbornness

Stubbornness is a common challenge with dementia. Fighting against losing independence and resistance to the change in roles can lead to a need to hang on to some sense of control. Stubbornness can also be the result of the inability to process information. "You can't tell me it's time to brush my teeth." "I don't need a shower. I just took one yesterday." "I can manage my own medication!" [15].

Spitting

They may no longer recognize the appropriate time and place for spitting. The person may not be swallowing as often and not know how to handle the excessive saliva in their mouth. It can also be a form of combative behavior expressing their anger or frustration [16]. Spitting can come in the form of spitting on the sidewalk, spitting out food, or spitting at someone.

Sundowning

Sundowning is a term used for changes in behavior that occur in the evening around dusk [17]. There may be an increase in behaviors or confusion as the late afternoon/evening or darkness approaches due to disturbance to the person's body clock due to the dementia. This can be particularly challenging during a time or season change. Sundowning can increase behaviors such as aggression, fear, and restlessness. Up to 66% of people with a dementia diagnosis will experience sundowning behaviors [18].

Taking Things

People with dementia may be driven to search for things that they perceive as missing or simply taking things that they think are theirs. This is also referred to as "shopping." They may think that the purse hanging on the back of a chair in a restaurant is their purse. You may find them wearing your glasses that you left in the bathroom even though your prescription is different or they don't wear glasses. They may take someone's sweater not because they need a sweater, but because they want to hold something or they desire the softness. There may be no identifiable reason—they just do it. Taking things is a common behavior and one that should be treated with sensitivity [19].

When reviewing all these potential behaviors, the most important thing to remember is that your loved one is your loved one even though they are behaving differently. As the caregiver, learning to manage behaviors can help to preserve the relationship. Embracing these changes may help with day-to-day living. Always remember, you did not sign up to be a caregiver. The person you are caring for did not sign up to have dementia.

Navigating this journey will be frustrating for both of you.

References

1. Dementia related behaviors. Alzheimer's Association; 2021. https://www.alz.org/media/documents/alzheimers-dementia-related-behaviors-ts.pdf.
2. Oxford English Dictionary. Aggression. In: oed.com dictionary. https://www.oed.com/search/dictionary/?scope=Entries&q=aggression. Accessed 26 Mar 2024.
3. Oxford English Dictionary. Anger. In: oed.com dictionary. https://www.oed.com/search/dictionary/?scope=Entries&q=anger. Accessed 26 Mar 2024.
4. Oxford English Dictionary. Anxiety. In: oed.com dictionary. https://www.oed.com/search/dictionary/?scope=Entries&q=anxiety. Accessed 26 Mar 2024.
5. Oxford English Dictionary. Delusions. In: oed.com dictionary. https://www.oed.com/search/dictionary/?scope=Entries&q=delusions. Accessed 26 Mar 2024.
6. PACE quality monitoring & reporting guidance. Center of Medicare Services; 2021. www.cms.gov/files/document/pacequalitymonitoringandreportingguidancemarch2021.pdf.
7. Wandering. Alzheimer's Association. https://www.alz.org/help-support/caregiving/safety/wandering.
8. Understanding the stress response. 2020. https://www.health.harvard.edu/staying:healthy/understanding-the-stress-response.
9. Oxford English Dictionary. Hallucination. In: oed.com dictionary. https://www.oed.com/search/dictionary/?scope=Entries&q=hallucination. Accessed 26 Mar 2024.
10. Hallucinations. Cleveland Clinic health library. https://my.clevelandclinic.org/health/symptoms/23350-hallucinations.
11. Hallucinations and dementia. 2021. https://www.alzheimers.org.uk/about-dementia/symptoms-and-diagnosis/hallucinations.
12. What is hoarding disorder?. American Psychiatric Association; 2021. https://www.psychiatry.org/patients-families/hoarding-disorder/what-is-hoarding-disorder.
13. Hernandez A. Hyperorality. What is it, causes, treatment and more. Osmosis from Elsevier. https://www.osmosis.org/answers/hyperorality.
14. Sleep issues and sundowning. Alzheimer's Association. https://www.alz.org/help-support/caregiving/stages-behaviors/sleep-issues-sundowning.
15. Cramer L. Dealing with resistance to care, Alzheimer's Association Caregiver Tips & Tools. California Central Coast Chapter. https://www.alz.org/media/cacentral/dementia-care-41-dealing-with-resistance-to-care.pdf.
16. Kar SK, Pandey P, Singh N. Understanding the psychological underpinning of spitting: relevance in the context of COVID-19. Indian J Psychol Med. 2020;42(6):577–8. https://doi.org/10.1177/0253717620962429.
17. Sundowning (Changes in Behaviours at Dusk). 2023. https://www.dementiauk.org/information-and-support/health-advice/sundowning/
18. Khachiyants N, Trinkle D, Son SJ, Kim KY. Sundown syndrome in persons with dementia: an update. Psychiatry Investig. 2011;8(4):275–87. https://doi.org/10.4306/pi.2011.8.4.275. Epub 2011 Nov 4.
19. Do people with early dementia resort to stealing? Health Central LLC; 2020. https://www.healthcentral.com/article/people-dementia-alzheimers-beginning-stages-resort-stealing.

Chapter 5
Foundational Tips

Now that you have an understanding of dementia, we offer you three foundational tips as you design your caregiving blueprint and aim to provide sustainable care through the dementia journey. The goal of *These Three Things*, which is introduced in Chap. 7, is to look at a situation and provide you with three options of how you can respond. This chapter will provide you with foundational tips to assist you in putting *These Three Things* into action while utilizing three additional concepts: critical thinking, creativity, and flexibility.

Critical Thinking

Critical Thinking
The objective analysis and evaluation of an issue in order to form a judgment [1].

Critical thinking is about taking in all of the information and seeing the bigger picture. There are three components to critical thinking [2]:

1. **Analyzing the situation**—observing what is happening utilizing the 5 W's—who, what, when, where, and why.
2. **Forming an opinion**—taking that information and determining what options you have for action. What can you do to resolve this situation?
3. **Making a decision**—Based on the information you have, what is the best action to implement? If your first choice does not work, try something else. Don't give up after just one try.

© The Author(s), under exclusive license to Springer Nature Switzerland AG 2024
L. Jenkins et al., *These Three Things*,
https://doi.org/10.1007/978-3-031-69394-6_5

CRITICAL THINKING

PROBLEM + THINKING = SOLUTION

When in the midst of caregiving, these steps will often need to happen very quickly. You are living in the moment and need to keep moving forward. That bigger picture is a snapshot of the moment.

Scenario 1
Your family just finished eating dinner. The table has been cleared and everyone has left the kitchen except your mother. She is asking you what you are serving for dinner and does not believe you when you say that you've all just finished eating. Mom is refusing to get up until she eats. How do you use critical thinking in this situation?

Analyze the situation: What are the key pieces of information you need to resolve this situation? Find the information utilizing who, what, when, where, and why.

Who: Your mom
What: She will not get up from the table. Everyone has already left the room.
When: 6:30 PM (note time—later in evening possible sundowning behavior—see glossary) after the family, including your mom, has already eaten dinner.
Where: In the kitchen
Why: She forgot that she has eaten dinner

Things to consider: Is mom a diabetic? Is mom under/overweight? Does she have night time meds that cannot interact with food? Do I have additional activities handy to divert her attention? Does she often become increasingly confused at night? What is happening in the adjoining room? Is there someone nearby that can help me call her to another room?

Form an opinion: After answering the questions above, is there one that sticks out? Is it harmful for her to have more food? Will it bother her to remain at the table with a glass of water while you do the dishes? Can someone call her into the other room to watch TV with the grandchildren?

Make a decision: You decide that the best option to try would be to give her a glass of water and engage her in conversation as you wash the dishes. In this case, it works beautifully!

There will be situations when you have more time with this process. You gather information over several instances and analyze the effectiveness of the actions you took. The bigger picture captures multiple instances of the same behavior or event. This is called tracking behaviors and it identifies possible trends. Acknowledging trends and patterns will increase the tools that you have to make an appropriate decision. This will ultimately give you the opportunity to be preventative with the behavior versus reacting to the situation.

Scenario 2
You notice that your mom is refusing to leave the table after dinner on most nights. She is growing less accepting of the glass of water and distracting conversation while remaining at the table. She continues to want to eat again becoming more demanding of food.

Analyze the situation: Looking back over several nights of this situation, what are the key pieces of information you need to find a resolution? Find the information utilizing who, what, when, where, and why thinking back on the past week.

Who: Your mom and family
What: She will not get up from the table.
When: 5 out of 7 days after the family, including your mom, has already eaten dinner. The table has been cleared and the rest of the family has left the room.
Where: She's in the kitchen without her family or plates on the table.
Why: She forgot that she has eaten dinner.

Things to consider: All visual cues of having eaten have been removed. Mom did not leave with everyone else. She is growing more demanding of food.

Form an opinion: After answering the questions above, what patterns or trends come to mind? Knowing that mom is a diabetic, giving in to her demands for more food is not a good option. With the trends that we've identified, how can we be more preventative in our actions. Can mom leave the table with a family member? Can mom carry her plate to the sink on her way out of the kitchen? Can the table be cleared after she leaves the room?

Make a decision: Knowing that mom is unsteady, carrying her plate to the sink is not an option. You decide to enlist the help of a family member to assist her in getting up and going into the other room for an activity such as playing cards or watching TV before the plates are cleared from the table.

Creativity

Creativity
The use of your imagination, the ability to generate or recognize ideas, alternatives, or possibilities [3].

As we know with dementia, when you see one person with dementia, you've seen one person with dementia. There is no one-size-fits-all package to traveling the road of dementia. Everybody progresses at different rates and responds to situations differently. Everyone's personalities are different. What works one day, may not work the next. And what didn't work today, may work beautifully tomorrow. Therefore, keep being creative. Being able to use your imagination to generate new ideas is going to be important when caring for someone with dementia.

This concept can be difficult or scary for some. Some may look for concrete step-by-step instructions of how to handle every situation. However, those instructions do not exist. Some people may not feel that they are creative. Everyone has the ability to be creative. It does not need to be a big gesture, It is simply having the courage to open up your mind and try something different. Trying things that you have not seen or heard is the pathway to new possibilities.

How do you tap into your creative side? Try these three things:

1. **Doodle**—Grab a pen and blank sheet of paper and freely draw. This will get your hands moving and your brain focused on something else. That can be all it takes to trigger a new idea!
2. **Get moving**—Go for a walk. Put on your favorite song and dance. This releases endorphins which promote creative thinking.
3. **Talk to someone**—This is a great way to switch up your thought process. You can talk over the specific situation with someone you trust bouncing ideas off each other. Interacting with someone new can promote learning things and introducing new ways of thinking.

Creativity paired with critical thinking will assist you with caring for your person with dementia. Adding those concepts to *These Three Things* will ignite a world of additional possibilities.

Flexibility
Flexibility is the willingness to change or compromise [4].
   Flexibility is having patience.

Flexibility is the final foundational tip to consider when implementing *These Three Things*. Everyone has expectations of how we think things will or should go.

Life does not work that way. When you are caring for someone with dementia, it is even more likely that your plan will not go as expected. Dementia is unpredictable.

Being flexible does not come easily for everyone.

If you struggle with being flexible, try *These Three Things*.

1. Take a deep breath and count to ten.
2. Shake off the preconceived notions of outcomes. Literally shake it off—shake your hands, your head, your hips, and visualize those notions flying off.
3. Be aware of your self-talk. Say out loud.
   "I did not sign up for this. Neither did my loved one."
   "This is a moment in time and it will pass."
   "This idea didn't work. What can I try next."

As the saying goes, "When the plan doesn't work, change the plan, not the goal" [5]. We must always keep our eyes focused on the goal of providing care for the person with dementia. Being flexible in that plan allows you to bend without breaking.

We've provided you with three foundational tips to assist you in putting *These Three Things* into action. Before we finally introduce *These Three Things*, we have a few more techniques to help you succeed in using them.

References

1. Oxford English Dictionary. Critical thinking. In. oed.com dictionary. https://www.oed.com/search/dictionary/?scope=Entries&q=critical++thinking. Accessed 26 Mar 2024.
2. Margot Note Consulting LLC. Three levels of critical thinking. 2020. https://www.margotnote.com/blog/2020/06/01/critical-thinking.
3. Oxford English Dictionary. Creativity. In: oed.com dictionary. https://www.oed.com/search/dictionary/?scope=Entries&q=creativity. Accessed 26 Mar 2024.
4. Oxford English Dictionary. Flexibility. In: oed.com dictionary. https://www.oed.com/search/dictionary/?scope=Entries&q=flexibility. Accessed 26 Mar 2024.
5. Author unknown. https://www.insightoftheday.com.

Chapter 6
Techniques

When caring for someone with dementia, there are six mainstay techniques that when mastered will help you on your journey. These can be adapted to any situation. While they look very simple, you will be challenged along your journey. Using these techniques in the non-dementia world may seem awkward and uncomfortable. But when focusing on the person with dementia, they take on new and helpful meanings. As you master these techniques over time, they will become automatic. Don't be too hard on yourself while you are learning these techniques. Dementia is forgiving.

Technique #1: Do Not Argue

This is an argument that you will lose every single time. The person with dementia has lost the ability to reason [1]. They can only see their perspective or may have forgotten the situation which you are discussing. To them time and place become blurred. Other times, it is an issue of control or trying to hold on to their independence. Everything is slipping away from them, but they have this moment to hold onto.

Another way to look at it is that if you enter in an argument with them, you walk away angry. The person you are caring for walks away and forgets that the argument ever took place. Though it is easy to know why you should not argue, this three letter word is the hard part—**HOW?**

If you are faced with not arguing, try *These Three Things*:

1. Take a deep breath and be willing to not be right.
2. Accept the fact that it truly does not matter who is right and who is wrong. You are looking for a positive interaction.

© The Author(s), under exclusive license to Springer Nature
Switzerland AG 2024
L. Jenkins et al., *These Three Things*,
https://doi.org/10.1007/978-3-031-69394-6_6

3. If you cannot let it go, literally walk away, slowly count to ten, re-enter the room
   and try another approach to the situation.

Technique #2: Enter Their Reality

It is common with dementia that the person's reality is not ours. People with dementia travel back in time as their mind is erased of the present. They may have a false belief or think something totally implausible. That's okay. Accept it. If it does not create any danger, join them in that moment. This will not cause them more confusion. In fact, this action can create calm and comfort. If your mom thinks that she is a singer at a nightclub, let her sing applauding her when she is done. If your dad thinks that you are his father or his brother, focus on the connection and not the title. Though it is easy to know why you should enter their reality, this three letter word is the hard part—**HOW?**

If you are faced with entering their reality, try *These Three Things*:

1. Listen. Engage in conversation. Don't assume that you know where their reality is in that moment.
2. Don't challenge or correct them.
3. Take a deep breath and play along with them validating their reality.

Technique #3: Five Words or Less

The pathways of the brain deteriorate making it harder to follow along with conversation. The person with dementia may only pick up three to five words or hold on to the last thing that you said [2]. They may take every word or phrase that you use literally. Increased words can lead to increased confusion and agitation. At the same time, using simple clear statements with five words or less can increase understanding and cooperation.

Though it is easy to know why you should use five words or less, this three letter word is the hard part—**HOW?**

If you are faced with using five words or less, try *These Three Things*:

1. Think before you speak. What were you going to say and how can you take that down to five words or less.
2. Offer directions one step at a time. "Unbutton your shirt." "Lift your arms." The next time you brush your teeth, talk yourself through the activity equating each action to offering one step at a time.
3. Practice using five words or less in everyday life when not providing care. For example, when discussing what vegetable to serve with dinner, break "Should we have peas or carrots for dinner tonight?" down to "Peas or carrots?"

Technique #4: Mirror Image

As the disease progresses, a person with dementia will forget how to accomplish everyday tasks. Things that were easy and done without thought will become a mystery. What is this shiny thing next to my plate? What am I supposed to do with it? Brush my teeth? What does that mean? By you completing a task at the same time, they can replicate the action just like watching themselves in a mirror.

Though it is easy to know why mirroring an action is helpful, this three letter word is the hard part—**HOW?**

If you are faced with mirroring an image, try *These Three Things*:

1. Sit directly across or stand directly in front of them
2. Show positive body language—maintain eye contact to ensure that they are watching you, offer positive reinforcement by nodding your head
3. Move slowly when completing the task step by step

Technique #5: Spaced Retrieval

Spaced retrieval is an evidenced-based technique that uses procedural memory to help people recall information [2, 3]. This is a valuable technique to use with someone who is asking a question over and over again. Confusion and worry that can be created by the memory loss can be eased with the use of the written word and gentle reminders. For example, you help your mom with her shower every Tuesday and Thursday. She starts to call you repeatedly asking when you are coming over to help her shower. You write the answer to the question on two post-it notes sticking one on the bathroom mirror and one by the phone. The next time your mom calls with that question, gently remind her to look at the note. The hope is that with repetition, this will become a new memory embedded in the brain. When she thinks of the question, she will be able to self-direct to the note and eventually recall the answer on her own. The repeated calls will stop. This technique can be adapted using pictures if the person cannot or has lost the ability to read.

Though it is easy to know spaced retrieval works, this three letter word is the hard part—**HOW?**

If you are faced with using space retrieval, try *These Three Things*:

1. Write only the answer to the question they are asking in large bold print with a contrasting ink using five words or less.
2. Place it in an area that is visible to the person.
3. Continue to direct them to the note while answering the question with the same wording until the new memory is created.

Technique #6: Therapeutic Truths

Ideally, we tell the truth all of the time; however, when you have dementia and are unable to reason or remember is it always helpful? A therapeutic truth is a statement that is untrue to preserve and protect the person with dementia's reality. It provides reassurance and comfort. For example, if your 84-year-old wife asks where her dad is, you can say that he is at work and will be home soon. Although her dad has passed away, reminding her of that fact subjects her to reliving the grief as if it is new every time.

If your dad will not leave the house for a necessary doctor's appointment, you can tell him that you are going out for lunch. This is an example of using a therapeutic truth for the greater good.

Though it is easy to understand why a therapeutic truth can be necessary, this three letter word is the hard part—**HOW?**

If you are faced with using a therapeutic truth, try *These Three Things*:

1. Keep it simple. There is no need to create an elaborate storyline.
2. Give yourself permission to tell a fib.
3. Match the story to the person making it believable.

While these six techniques can be adapted to any situation, they may not work every time. What works today may not work tomorrow. And what does not work today may go beautifully tomorrow. There is great variation in when and how often they will work. Don't lose hope. Be creative and flexible. Do what is comfortable for you.

References

1. What is dementia? https://www.scie.org.uk/dementia/.
2. Carpenter SK, Pan SC, Butler AC. The science of effective learning with spacing and retrieval practice. Nat Rev Psychol. 2022;1:496–511. https://doi.org/10.1038/s44159-022-00089-1.
3. Small JA, Cochrane D. Spaced retrieval and episodic memory training in Alzheimer's disease. Clin Interv Aging. 2020;15:519–36. https://doi.org/10.2147/CIA.S242113.

Chapter 7
These Three Things

All of the information we have shared so far in the previous chapters has given you the overview of dementia to utilize the most important tool – *These Three Things*. In this chapter, you will find examples of behaviors that are common in dementia but more importantly three things to manage those behaviors.

Activities of Daily Living (ADLs)

When faced with the challenge of *refusing to brush their teeth*, try *These Three Things*.

1. Use mirror image—brush your teeth, too.
2. Put on music and brush to the beat.
3. Make sure the toothpaste is not too minty.
   They may not be able to communicate that the toothpaste is burning his mouth.

When faced with the challenge of *being afraid to take a shower*, try *These Three Things*.

1. Calmly explain step by step what you are doing as you do it.
   "It's time to take shower."
   "Let's take off your shoes."
   "Let's take off your socks."
2. Play their favorite or calming music.
3. Prepare the room before taking the person into the bathroom.
   Do you have all of the supplies that you need?
   Check the temperature of the room. Is it warm enough?

© The Author(s), under exclusive license to Springer Nature
Switzerland AG 2024
L. Jenkins et al., *These Three Things*,
https://doi.org/10.1007/978-3-031-69394-6_7

When faced with the challenge of *refusing to take a shower* try *These Three Things*.

1. Ask yourself, "Who is this bothering?"
     As people age, they don't need to bathe as often.
     The water and soap can dry out the skin.
     Different cultures view bathing differently.
2. Use a therapeutic truth
     "We're having company today."
     "You have an appointment."
3. Try again at a better time

When faced with the challenge of *providing nail care* try *These Three Things*.

1. Provide care on a routine basis
2. Make it fun
     Have a spa day
     Soak nails in warm water
     Use scented lotion
     Play music
3. Offer a distraction
     Have someone else sit and talk with them
     Lay a towel over their arms
     Put on the TV

When faced with the challenge of *disrobing* try *These Three Things*.

1. Ensure that clothes fit comfortably
2. Dress in clothes that are harder for them to remove
     Overalls
     Jumpsuits
     Put clothes on backwards
3. Redirect into activity or conversation

When faced with the challenge of *getting dressed*, try *These Three Things*.

1. Use five words or less
     "Put on your shirt."
     "Pull up your pants."
2. Offer to help.
     "Can I help you?"
     "Let me see."
3. Simplify the clothing
     Pants with an elastic waist
     Shoes with Velcro
     Shirts with a large neck opening

When faced with the challenge of *not changing clothes*, try *These Three Things*.

1. Simplify the choices of clothes in the closet
     Remove items that do not fit, are not appropriate for the season or are soiled.
     Hang outfits together on one hanger.
2. Offer two choices
     "Blue Shirt or Red Shirt?"
3. Use a therapeutic truth
     "You have an appointment."
     "We're expecting company."

When faced with the challenge of *not dressing appropriately for the weather* try *These Three Things*.

1. Ask yourself, "Who is this bothering?"
2. Remove access to seasonal clothes, shoes, outerwear
     Take winter coat out of the closet in the Spring
     Remove short sleeved shirts from their dresser in the Fall
3. Use a therapeutic truth
     "Here is a gift."
     "Does this fit?"
     "There's a stain on that."

When faced with the challenge of *refusing to put on their coat* try *These Three Things*.

1. Hand them their coat
2. Use mirror image and put on your coat
3. Ask yourself, "Is it necessary?"
    Will they be getting into a warm car?
    Will there be any harm if a coat is not worn.

When faced with the challenge of *maintaining independence* try *These Three Things*.

1. Set them up for success by offering simple steps and limiting choices.
2. Adapt task to their ability
    Velcro instead of buttons
    Pull-on pants instead of zippers
    Crock-pot instead of oven
3. Look at adaptable equipment/devices.
    Cup with a lid
    Plate with a rim
    Grab bars by the toilet

Behaviors

When faced with the challenge of *communication struggles*, try *These Three Things*.

1. Use five words or less
    "Come with me."
    "It's time to eat."
    "Can you help me?"
2. Don't argue
    This is an argument that you will never win.
3. Pay attention to your nonverbal communication
    Maintain eye contact.
    Keep your arms open instead of crossed.
    Be aware of your facial expressions

When faced with the challenge of *repeating stories or questions* try *These Three Things*.

1. Enter their reality.
2. Use spaced retrieval.
   Write the answer to the question on a piece of paper or notecard.
   Direct to look at the paper/card every time the question is asked.
3. Redirect into an activity or another topic.

When faced with the challenge of *calling you repeatedly* try *These Three Things*.

1. Use the same statement every time they call
   "You are safe."
   "Everything is fine."
   "I'll check on you soon."
2. Be proactive. Call them on a routine/scheduled basis
3. Set up a reassuring voicemail message that allows you to let the call go to voicemail
   "Mom—Everything is fine."
   "I'm on the other line."
   "I'll call you soon."

When faced with the challenge of *arguing* try *These Three Things*.

1. Change the focus
   Provide a distraction
   Ask a question
2. Live in their world
   If they think its raining, it is raining.
   If they think its 1975, it is 1975.
3. Take a break and walk away

When faced with the challenge of *hoarding (non-food)*, try *These Three Things*.

1. Create a fidget box or drawer for rummaging. Fill it with items of interest or importance to the person.
2. Use a therapeutic truth to promote removing items from the home.
   "We're donating these items."
   "A family needs this."
   "Can I borrow these?"
3. Limit what you bring into the home.
   Sort mail before bringing it in.
   Stop or reduce newspaper delivery.

When faced with the challenge of *preventing aggressive behavior* try *These Three Things*.

1. Create a calm environment
   Play soft music
   Limit stimulation
   Be aware of what is on the television.
2. Enter their reality
3. Be mindful of your attitude and communication
   Remember that he/she will mirror your behaviors and emotions
   Validate their feelings/experiences

When faced with the challenge of *managing aggression*, try *These Three Things*.

1. Remain calm
   Remember that they will mirror your behaviors and emotions.
   Take a few deep breaths.
   Don't react aggressively.
2. Attempt to redirect/distract
   Ask a question about a different topic.
   Ring the doorbell/phone.
   Drop something like a book, a pillow or your keys.
   Talk softly.
3. Create a safe place for you. It is okay to walk away.

When faced with the challenge of *difficult behaviors in public*, try *These Three Things*.

1. Educate those around you with a button or business card that has a pre-printed statement that states "My loved one has dementia. Please be patient and understanding."
2. Be proactive, not reactive.
   Be aware of triggers.
   Make sure basic needs are met before leaving.
3. Be aware of your surroundings.
   Sit in a quiet area.
   Avoid overstimulation.

When faced with the challenge of *public sexual behaviors*, try *These Three Things*.

1. Offer privacy
2. Don't overreact
3. Don't shame the person

When faced with the challenge of *inappropriate touching of others*, try *These Three Things*.

1. Give them something to hold
2. Redirect them to an activity, to a chore, or to look at something in the room
3. Watch your positioning—stand an arm length's away, don't turn your back

When faced with the challenge of *inappropriate language*, try *These Three Things*.

1. Don't overreact.
2. Focus on the emotion.
3. Provide a distraction.
   Change the subject.
   Offer a snack.
   Exclaim with a big reaction "Look at that!" and point at something.

When faced with the challenge of *anxiety/fear*, try *These Three Things*.

1. Provide reassurance in a quiet calm voice.
   "You are safe here."
   "I'll stay here with you."
   "Sorry you feel this way."
2. Provide a calm environment.
   Decrease noise.
   Move to another room.
   Limit stimulation.
3. Distract with an activity such as
   Singing a song
   Watch TV
   Going for a walk

When faced with the challenge of *the person being afraid*, try *These Three Things*.

1. Provide reassurance with words and touch.
2. Focus on the emotion as they may not be able to tell you why they are afraid.
3. Provide a comfort item.
   Baby doll
   Stuffed animal
   Soft blanket

When faced with the challenge of *hallucinations*, try *These Three Things*.

1. Don't argue. It is real to them.
      Smash the spider.
      Spray the bugs.
      Use the umbrella.
2. Don't dismiss their emotions/experience
3. If they are not frightened by it, embrace it.
      Welcome the friend to the table.
      Acknowledge the puppy.

When faced with the challenge of *delusions*, try *These Three Things*.

1. Don't take offense if accused of something. Remember this is the disease.
2. Recognize your loved one's feelings and offer a simple response.
3. Provide a distraction.
      Introduce them to an activity.
      Sing a song.
      Do something active such as going for a walk.
      Give them a comfort item to hold.

When faced with the challenge of *paranoia*, try *These Three Things*.

1. Provide reassurance.
      Focus on the emotion—they are afraid.
      Affirm that he/she is safe.
2. Enter their reality.
      "I'm going to lock the door."
      "We're safe."
      "He can't get in here."
3. Do not argue or attempt to reason.

When faced with the challenge of *shadowing*, try *These Three Things*.

1. Distract with an activity.
2. Offer reassurance that they are safe.
3. Utilize spaced retrieval.
    A picture of you to hold.
    A note that you'll be right back.

When faced with the challenge of *the person making false accusation*, try *These Three Things*.

1. Be aware of your reaction.
    Do not argue with them.
    Do not overreact.
    Watch your nonverbal communication.
2. Side with them using a therapeutic truth.
    "These are bad things."
    "Don't worry."
    "I'll take care of it."
3. Provide a distraction such as
    Offering food and/or drink
    Pretend to receive a phone call
    Turn on music

When faced with the challenge of *continuous pacing*, try *These Three Things*.

1. Ask yourself, "Who is this bothering?"
    If there is not a fall risk or they are not overly tired, let them go.
    Make sure there is a clear path to walk.
    Ensure that the environment is safe.
2. Offer other movement
    Porch swing
    Rocking chair
    Dancing
3. Provide a distraction
    Turn on the TV
    Offer them a magazine or photo album
    Give them something to hold

When faced with the challenge of *sundowning*, try *These Three Things*.

1. Maintain a routine.
    Eat dinner at the same time.
    Go to bed at the same time.
2. Plan for it—be proactive, not reactive.
    Can you identify his/her pattern of behavior?
    When is the next full moon?
3. Be aware of the environment.
    Dim the lights.
    Turn down the TV/Music volume.
    Talk softly.

When faced with the challenge of *a full moon*, try *These Three Things*.

1. Know when the full moon is occurring.
2. Track behaviors during full moons.
3. Prepare in advance for increased behaviors.
    Maintain routine and schedule.
    Limit stimulation.

When faced with the challenge of *spitting*, try *These Three Things*.

1. Give a cup or rag for them to spit into.
2. Give them something to put in their mouth.
    Sucker
    Gum
    Hard candy
3. Ask yourself, "Are they trying to communicate something?"
    Frustration
    Pain
    Illness

When faced with the challenge of *hyperorality (hyper oral)*, try *These Three Things*.

1. Offer them a safe food choice.
2. Remove items from the environment which could be confused for food or could be a choking hazard such as
   Poker chips
   Coins
   Fake fruit
   Styrofoam
3. Mirror image to have them open their mouth.

When faced with the challenge of *picking or scratching at skin*, try *These Three Things*.

1. Give them something to hold in their hands.
   Stress ball
   Blanket
   Book
2. Dress them in long sleeves, long pants, or cotton gloves.
3. Maintain personal hygiene.
   Keep nails trimmed.
   Apply lotion to moisturize skin.

When faced with the challenge of *not wanting to get in the car*, try *These Three Things*.

1. Play music from their youth and reminisce.
2. Enlist the help of someone else.
3. Use a Therapeutic Truth
   "We're meeting your grandson."
   "We can't be late."
   "I can't go alone."

When faced with the challenge of *not wanting to get out of the car*, try *These Three Things*.

1. Drive around the block and try again.
2. Enlist the help of someone else.
3. Use a therapeutic truth
     "Your daughter is waiting inside!"
     "We're going to a party!"
     "We can't be late."
     "Another car is behind us."

When faced with the challenge of *taking something that is not theirs*, try *These Three Things*.

1. Ask yourself—Who is it bothering?
2. Offer them a trade over-emphasizing that what you're offering is better.
     If they take your wallet, offer them a purse.
     If they take your water glass, offer them a fresh glass.
3. Divert their attention and remove the item.

When faced with the challenge of *thinking that something belongs to them that is not theirs*, try *These Three Things*.

1. Don't argue.
2. Distract them bygiving them something else.
     Changing the conversation.
     Offering them a trade.
3. Enter their reality. They'll eventually move on leaving the item behind.

Caregiving

When faced with the challenge of *accepting that your loved one has this disease*, try *These Three Things*.

1. Educate yourself.
2. Allow yourself to grieve.
3. Seek additional support as needed
     Counseling
     A caregiver support group

When faced with the challenge of *not recognizing you*, try *These Three Things*.

1. Enter their reality—whoever they think you are, you are!
2. Leave the room and re-enter.
3. Avoid quizzing them and introduce yourself.

When faced with the challenge of *feeling guilty about taking time for yourself*, try *These Three Things*.

1. Talk about your feelings—in a support group, with a friend, clergy, or therapist.
2. Stop negative self-talk by identifying three positive facts about yourself/situation.
3. Spend time reflecting on the goals and expectations that you have for yourself. Are they reasonable? How can you adapt them to set yourself up for success?

When faced with the challenge of *feeling like I'm going to lose it*, try *These Three Things*.

1. Pause and take ten slow deep breaths. Realize that you are doing the best that you can.
2. Play your favorite song and loudly sing along.
3. Sit down and drink a cup of coffee/tea.

When faced with the challenge of *managing the long-term stress of caregiving*, try *These Three Things*.

1. Acknowledge it—It is okay to feel stressed. Just like your loved one didn't sign up for this, neither did you.
2. Find outlets of happiness.
     Listen to music.
     Eat dessert.
     Buy yourself flowers.
     Connect with a friend.
3. Maintain your own healthy habits.
     Exercise.
     Eat healthy meals.
     Get enough sleep.

When faced with the challenge of *you being sick*, try *These Three Things*.

1. Enlist the help of others. It is okay!
2. Maintain routine as much as possible.
3. Provide activities for them such as:
     Fidget box
     Word puzzles
     Folding towels

When faced with the challenge of *needing to be away from the person*, try *These Three Things…*

1. Prepare and educate the person caring for them especially about routine and elopement risk.
2. Attempt to have someone come into their home vs them going somewhere else.
3. Give short notice of the upcoming separation to your loved one to minimize anxiety and additional behaviors.

When faced with the challenge of *explaining dementia to young children*, try *These Three Things…*

1. Use words that they would understand.
2. Buy them a book about dementia.
3. Reassure them that love remains
   Even if the person doesn't remember us, we still remember them.
   The person will be okay.

When faced with the challenge of *family members not agreeing on care*, try *These Three Things.*

1. Remember that while you are all different, you are all there for the same reason.
2. Keep communication open establishing ground rules.
   No raised voices
   No name calling
   Avoid triangulation
3. Find a neutral party or professional to facilitate the discussion.

When faced with the challenge of *needing help from others*, try *These Three Things*.

1. Remember that you are human and you can't do it all.
2. Trust that people want to help you.
3. Be specific when asking for or accepting help.

When faced with the challenge of *looking for community resources*, try *These Three Things…*

1. Call your county's office on aging
2. Contact your local Alzheimer's Association (or other disease specific organizations)
3. Talk with those around you—neighbors, friends, medical team.

Change

When faced with the challenge of *change*, try *These Three Things*.

1. Don't notify them of the upcoming change too far in advance.
2. Offer emotional support.
   Provide reassurance.
   Be patient.
3. Allow extra time to adapt to the change.

When faced with the challenge of *the change of seasons*, try *These Three Things*.

1. Maintain their routine.
2. Be aware of the increased elopement risk.
3. Remove access to seasonal clothes, shoes, and outerwear.
     Take winter coat out of the closet in the Spring.
     Remove short sleeved shirts from their dresser in the Fall.

When faced with the challenge of *daylight savings time*, try *These Three Things*…

1. Begin to either move bedtime up or back by 15 min a week for 3–4 weeks prior to the time change.
2. Be aware of increased elopement risk.
3. Maintain their routine.

When faced with the challenge of *moving to a new living environment*, try *These Three Things*.

1. Set up rooms to the way they had it before.
2. Maintain routine as change can ignite behaviors.
3. Recognize that this is an elopement/wandering risk.

When faced with the challenge of *transitioning from one activity to the next*, try *These Three Things...*

1. Provide a distraction.
   Ring the doorbell.
   Have someone call their name from a different room.
2. Exit the room and return a few minutes later to try again.
3. Ask yourself if the activity is necessary at this moment.

When faced with the challenge of *leaving a room to go to another*, try *These Three Things...*

1. Provide a distraction.
   Ring the doorbell.
   Start singing.
   Turn on the TV or music in a different room.
2. Use a simple statement.
   "Come help me."
   "Come with me."
3. Have someone else try.

When faced with the challenge of *a loved one passing away*, try *These Three Things.*

1. Determine if it is necessary for them to know.
2. Don't correct them if they talk about the person as if they are still alive.
3. Follow their lead in grieving. Recognize that their grieving process may be different than would be expected due to the dementia.

Medical

When faced with the challenge of *being asked "What is wrong with me?,"* try *These Three Things*.

1. Be honest—
     "You have a medical diagnosis."
     "We will talk to doctor."
     "I'm taking care of you."
2. Focus on the person's positive attributes.
3. If question is being asked repeatedly, change your approach.
     Divert into an activity.
     Introduce another topic.
     Use humor—"I know what's wrong. We're O-L-D."

When faced with the challenge of *their sadness or depression*, try *These Three Things*.

1. Be present with them.
     Offer verbal reassurance.
     Give them a hug or hold their hand.
     Sit with them.
2. Consult your medical provider—depression is treatable.
3. Encourage exposure to natural light or light sources
     Go outside even for just a few minutes
     Open the curtains.

When faced with the challenge of *not wanting to take medication*, try *These Three Things*.

1. Hand it to them, don't ask.
2. Mirror the action by taking your pills together.
3. Consult with their primary care provider.
     Can the medication be given in a different form?
     Can we reduce the number of pills?

When faced with the challenge of *the person being sick*, try *These Three Things*.

1. Offer reassurance that they are ok.
2. Be aware of increased confusion and/or behaviors.
3. Keep common supplies such as tissues, fluids, and a bucket in line of sight.

When faced with the challenge of *the person having a Urinary Tract Infection*, try *These Three Things*.

1. Be aware of rapid onset of
    Increased confusion
    Unusual behaviors
    Unsteadiness
2. Increase fluid intake
3. Be prepared for increased incontinence

When faced with the challenge of *suspecting they are in pain, but they can't communicate it* try *These Three Things*...

1. Ask yourself is there something else going on.
    Are clothing/socks/shoes too tight?
    Are there rough clothing tags?
    Are there any minor cuts or rashes?
2. Medicate appropriately.
    Over-the-counter medications
    Prescribed medications
    Communicate with medical provider as needed
3. Remember that aches and pains they've had will remain after a dementia diagnosis.

When faced with the challenge of *going to appointments*, try *These Three Things*.

1. Plan appointments at a time that is good for them.
     Are they a morning person?
     Do they like to sleep in later?
     Are they more tired by the end of the week?
     Are there already two appointments scheduled that week?
2. Don't give them advanced notice.
3. Alert the staff at the office of the dementia diagnosis.

When faced with the challenge of *a dentist appointment*, try *These Three Things*.

1. Consult with the dentist. Is this still necessary?
     What was their prior habit?
     Do they need the full exam or just a cleaning?
     What is the best plan of treatment for them?
2. Provide routine mouth care
3. Provide extra support
     Sit with them during treatment
     Provide something for them to hold

When faced with the challenge of *a podiatry appointment*, try *These Three Things*.

1. Consult with the podiatrist. How often is this necessary?
2. Give them something to hold during the appointment.
3. Provide routine foot care.

Nutrition

When faced with the challenge of *keeping them hydrated*, try *These Three Things…*

1. Use mirror image and have a drink with them Cheers!
2. Offer options other than water.
   Popsicles
   Jello
   Water-based fruits such as watermelon
   Soups
3. Hand them the glass.
   Don't ask if they want it.
   "Here's your drink."

When faced with the challenge of *initiating eating*, try *These Three Things.*

1. Use mirror image
   Sit across from them at the table.
   They'll see you eating and mirror your actions.
2. Simplify the plate
   Place one or two food items on the plate at a time.
   Use a smaller plate.
3. Use a bright solid colored plate such as red to provide a contrast between the food and the plate.

When faced with the challenge of *forgetting that they've eaten*, try *These Three Things…*

1. Offer a small snack or glass of water
2. Redirect into an activity not food related
3. Change their environment—move to a different room

When faced with the challenge of *hoarding food*, try *These Three Things*.

1. Remove it—Have someone distract them while you are disposing of the food.
2. Use therapeutic truths
    Let's donate it!
    There's a Food Drive.
3. Look at what is being brought into the home.
    Only bring in small quantities of food.
    Choose food with a long shelf life.

When faced with the challenge of *pocketing food*, try *These Three Things*.

1. Provide step-by-step instructions on swallowing
    "Keep chewing."
    "Swallow your food."
    Demonstrate swallowing.
2. Be prepared with napkins to dispose of unwanted food.
3. Offer liquids with each bite.
    If this behavior continues, reach out to your medical provider.

Safety

When faced with the challenge of *elopement risk*, try *These Three Things*.

1. Provide supervision being aware of exit seeking behaviors at all times
2. Create Distractions
    Hang a stop sign on back of the door
    Place a black mat in front of door
    Set a fidget box/table beside door
3. Be aware of changes in routine/environment
    Visiting family
    New caregiving staff
    Moving to a new home or room

When faced with the challenge of *an elopement*, try *These Three Things*.

1. Time is of the essence.
   Call out their name.
   Conduct a thorough search of the house and yard including closets, basements, and sheds.
2. Call the Police/911.
3. Keep an updated picture on your phone.

When faced with the challenge of *smoking that has become unsafe*, try *These Three Things*.

1. Remove cigarettes, ash trays, and other smoking-related items from their environment.
2. Consult with their provider about nicotine replacement (patch, gum).
3. Be sure safety measures are in place.
   Spray fire retardant on furniture, bedding, and other areas.
   Ensure that fire alarms are working properly.

When faced with the challenge of *smoking in an inappropriate/non-smoking environment*, try *These Three Things*.

1. Offer them something to hold and/or put in their mouth such as a lollipop or straw.
2. Offer a beverage.
3. Focus on the emotion—"I know this stinks. This is so hard."

When faced with the challenge of *unsafe cooking*, try *These Three Things…*

1. Remove the knobs and/or disable the stove.
2. Offer finger foods or other foods that don't require cooking.
3. Cook with the person.

When faced with the challenge of *driving that has become worrisome* try *These Three Things…*

1. Physically remove the keys from the home and/or disable the car.
2. Blame someone else such as the doctor or an out-of-town relative.
3. Focus on what they need.
   Take them to the store on a regular basis or have groceries delivered.
   Enjoy an afternoon drive

When faced with the challenge of *falls*, try *These Three Things*.

1. Keep walking pathways clear.
   Remove throw rugs.
   Secure cords
2. Check for safe shoes/footwear.
   Avoid backless shoes and high heels.
   Wear sturdy tennis shoes
3. Report falls to medical provider for medication review.

When faced with the challenge of *using ambulatory assistive devices*, try *These Three Things*...

1. Encourage use of device.
    "Here's your walker!"
    Avoid quizzing—"Aren't you forgetting something?"
    Keep the device where they can see it.
2. Decorate/personalize it with their name and colors/items they enjoy.
3. Utilize spaced retrieval putting notes in places such as where they normally sit, on the door or on the device saying.
    "Take me!"
    "Doctor's orders. Please use."
    "Don't forget your walker."

When faced with *the challenge of mismanaging finances*, try *These Three Things*...

1. Limit access to money.
    Remove check book.
    Cancel credit cards or reduce available credit limit.
2. Set bills up on direct payment or have bills forwarded to yourself.
3. Give the person a small amount of cash in small bills.

When faced with the challenge of *safe proofing your home from chemicals*, try *These Three Things*.

1. Place a warning sticker on the bottles and lock them up.
2. Buy natural-based cleaning products.
3. Fill a spray bottle with water.

When faced with the challenge of *repeatedly calling 911*, try *These Three Things*.

1. Use spaced retrieval with notes that state:
    Call your family first at 123-456-7890.
    You are safe.
2. Provide frequent phone calls offering verbal reassurance that they are safe.
3. Get them an ERS—Emergency Response System (consider having you be the first contact rather than immediately dispatching 911).

When faced with the challenge of *struggling to care for a pet*, try *These Three Things…*

1. Try automatic equipment for pet care.
    Automatic feeder.
    Self-cleaning litter box.
2. Use a therapeutic truth.
    "Pets are not permitted here."
    "I'm allergic to dogs."
3. Utilize an electronic or stuffed pet.

When faced with the challenge of *unnecessarily adjusting the thermostat*, try *These Three Things*.

1. Hide it from site or disguise it by covering it with a
    Plastic cover
    Picture
    Wall hanging
2. Consider changing to a digital thermostat.
3. Check their clothing—Do they need to wear heavier or lighter clothes?

Sleep

When faced with the challenge of *wanting to go to bed too early*, try *These Three Things*.

1. Encourage physical activity.
     Take a walk.
     Get up and dance.
     Do seated exercises.
2. Change the environment.
3. Keep lights on as much as possible until bed time.

When faced with the challenge of *not sleeping through the night*, try *These Three Things…*

1. Maintain healthy sleep habits.
     Only wear pajamas at night.
     Use the bed only for sleeping.
     Go to bed and wake up at the same time.
     Ensure that all needs are met—use the bathroom, small nightlight for safety, small snack before bed.
2. Limit fluids beginning 4 hours before bedtime.
3. Discuss sleep concerns with provider as medications can impact sleep.

When faced with the challenge of *having their days and nights mixed up*, try *These Three Things…*

1. During the day.
     Maintain a routine.
     Avoid napping.
     Keep them active and engaged.
     Avoid caffeine after noon.
2. Keep lights on as much as possible until bedtime.
3. Maintain healthy sleep habits.
     Only wear pajamas at night.
     Use the bed only for sleeping.
     Go to bed and wake up at the same time.
     Ensure that all needs are met—use the bathroom, small nightlight for safety, small snack before met.

When faced with the challenge of *keeping your loved one safe while you're sleeping*, try *These Three Things…*

1. Use a baby monitor so that you can hear them.
2. Install a door alarm on their bedroom door and/or the front door.
3. Be open to ask for someone to come sit with them so that you can get a restful sleep.

Socializing

When faced with the challenge of *going to the hairdresser*, try *These Three Things*.

1. Educate hairdresser about dementia ahead of time.
2. Can accommodations be made?
    Can they come to the house?
    Schedule the appointment during a quiet time.
    Ask hairdresser to limit options.
3. Read their body language.
    Facing the mirror may provide positive stimulations (watching the process, having a conversation with the person they see).
    If facing the mirror becomes distressing (not recognizing the person they see), turn them away.
    Be aware that the hair dryer may be scary to the person.

When faced with the challenge of *attending a special event*, try *These Three Things*.

1. Have a plan—be proactive, not reactive.
    Adjust time as needed.
    Check out the venue ahead of time—parking situation, seating arrangements.
    Alert the host/hostess of the dementia diagnosis if appropriate.
2. Take a comfort item (pillow, picture book, blanket).
3. Don't leave them alone.
    Accompany them to the bathroom.
    Walk with them through the buffet line.

When faced with the challenge of *holiday celebrations*, try *These Three Things*.

1. Keep decorations simple and safe.
   Avoid blinking lights.
   Minimize decorations.
   Avoid rearranging furniture.
2. Watch for signs of over stimulation.
   Pacing
   Agitation
   Anxiety
3. Maintain routine as much as possible.

When faced with the challenge of *having visitors*, try *These Three Things*.

1. Plan the visit.
   Choose a good time of day.
   Have a simple activity planned.
   Make sure basic needs are met.
2. Prepare the visitor by educating them.
   Alert the visitor of what to expect.
   Tips for conversation.
3. Limit the length of the visit.

When faced with the challenge of *visiting in a facility*, try *These Three Things*.

1. Choose a good time of day.
   Check the activity calendar of the facility.
   Limit the length of the visit.
2. Choose a quiet area within the facility.
3. Bring a treat or comfort item with you.

When faced with the challenge of *not having a meaningful visit*, try *These Three Things…*

1. Set realistic expectations remembering that they have a disease.
2. Go into the visit with a prepared activity.
3. It is acceptable to end the visit earlier than you expected.

When faced with the challenge of *leaving the facility after a visit*, try *These Three Things…*

1. Plan your visit around mealtime so that you can walk them to the dining room and get them set to eat.
2. Use a therapeutic truth.
    "I have to check something."
    "I need the bathroom."
    "I'll be right back."
3. Notify staff that you are leaving and ask them to assist you.

Toileting

When faced with the challenge of *being unable to verbalize need to use the bathroom*, try *These Three Things…*

1. Watch for nonverbal cues
    Removing or pulling at clothing
    Fidgeting
    Wandering around house
2. Place a sign/picture of toilet on the bathroom door
3. Maintain a routine/schedule encouraging use of the bathroom every 2 hours

When faced with the challenge of *not wanting to use the bathroom*, try *These Three Things...*

1. Make a schedule and encourage use of the bathroom every 2 hours
2. Use a therapeutic truth
    "We have an appointment."
    "A guest is coming!"
3. Make a simple statement
    "Come with me."
    "Let's go to the bathroom."

When faced with the challenge of *not accepting assistance with changing incontinence products*, try *These Three Things...*

1. Be sure that all supplies are within reach before you go into the bathroom.
2. Provide a distraction.
    Ask them to hold something.
3. Sing or hum a familiar song.

When faced with the challenge of *urinating in the inappropriately house*, try *These Three Things...*

1. Use spaced retrieval
    Place a sign on the bathroom door
    Place a picture of a toilet on the bathroom door
2. Follow a toileting schedule of every 2 or 3 hours
3. Remove tempting items such as fake trees and garbage cans

When faced with the challenge of *public urination*, try *These Three Things*.

1. Prepare for the outing
    Limit fluids before leaving
    Make sure they use the bathroom before going on the outing
    Take an extra set of clothes
2. Wear incontinence products when on outings
    Pull-ups
    Pads
3. Watch for nonverbal signs of having to use the restroom
    Pulling on pants
    Looking uncomfortable
    Searching for something

When faced with the challenge of _____, try *These Three Things.*

1. _____
   _____
   _____
2. _____
   _____
   _____
3. _____
   _____
   _____

Chapter 8
Taking Care of You

It is well documented through research that being a caregiver takes a toll on a person's health—physical, mental, emotional, social, spiritual, and financial. Research also shows that taking care of a person with dementia can lead to an even greater strain on a person's health than caring for people with other illnesses [1, 2]. In the world of caregiving, one can feel very overwhelmed focusing all their attention on the needs of the one for which they are caring. The caregiver's needs end up on the bottom of the "To Do List." As a result, the caregiver's health may suffer.

Caregivers often hear, "You should take time for yourself." "You need to take care of you." "If you don't take care of yourself, who will take care of Bob?" "Don't forget about you." The question the caregiver is left asking is, "How do I do that?" Let us show you that how.

A myth about self-care is that it must be a big event—potentially take a lot of time or cost money. Often when people think of self-care they think of massages, manicures, shopping sprees, and weekend escapes. These things are forms of self-care; but it is not always realistic to be able to incorporate those into a caregiver's life on a regular basis. Then, when we can't make it happen, we get frustrated and give up.

A different approach is to incorporate small self-care activities into our lives on a regular basis. Research has shown that these mini moments—or micro-practices as they are also called—can have a greater impact on our health than one or two BIG activities every year [3, 4]. Those moments are easier to achieve on a consistent basis and, therefore, our self-care tank is filled and energy is increased. This helps to keep motivation focused and positivity intact. Your drive to continue providing care also depends on taking care of you.

If you have *1 min for self-care*, try *These Three Things*:

1. Take five slow deep breaths.
2. List three things that you are grateful for in this moment.

© The Author(s), under exclusive license to Springer Nature
Switzerland AG 2024
L. Jenkins et al., *These Three Things*,
https://doi.org/10.1007/978-3-031-69394-6_8

3. Strike a power pose. Stand with your feet hip width apart. Make two fists and place them on your hips. Take in a deep breath while pushing your chest forward and pushing your shoulders back. Lift your chin. This may feel silly, but research shows that this will reduce cortisol (the stress hormone) and increase testosterone (the confidence hormone) [5]. Go ahead and unleash your inner superhero!

If you have *5 min for self-care*, try *These Three Things*:

1. Put on your favorite song and sing along loudly or dance around.
2. Complete a 5-4-3-2-1 Mindfulness Exercise. Take a few deep breaths. Look around you and identify

   (a) five things you can see
   (b) four things you can touch
   (c) three things you can hear
   (d) two things you can smell
   (e) one thing you can taste

3. Get a glass of water and drink it slowly.

If you have *15 min for self-care*, try *These Three Things*:

1. Make yourself a cup of tea or lemonade. Sit down and enjoy it!
2. Call a friend just to say hello.
3. Scroll through social media.

If you have *30 min for self-care and can't leave the house*, try *These Three Things*:

1. Do something creative!
   Write a poem.
   Doodle.
   Paint with watercolors.
2. Read a book.
3. Laugh! Put on funny videos or a classic TV comedy or a comedian.

If you have *30 min for self-care and you CAN leave the house*, try *These Three Things*...

1. Go for a walk in your neighborhood.
2. Go outside. Find a grassy spot, take your shoes off and stand in the grass. Look up at the clouds. Listen to the birds. Breathe in the fresh air.
3. Treat yourself to your favorite coffee or an ice cream cone.

If you have *1 h for self-care and you CAN leave the house*, try *These Three Things*...

1. Go to a park. Sit on a bench and people watch, Take a walk.
2. Go outside. Find a grassy spot, take your shoes off and stand in the grass. Look up at the clouds. Listen to the birds. Breathe in the fresh air.
3. Go for a drive. Listen to your favorite music or podcast. Enjoy the silence.

Even with these suggestions, self-care can be hard. We often know the healthy choices we can make and need to make, but we get stuck in following through and actually doing it. We're literally stuck sitting on the couch or standing in the kitchen because we've stopped moving and now we're so tired that we can't move. The self-induced pressure of completing our long "To Do" list is so heavy. We're too overwhelmed to take action. We just don't want to do it.

If you are *feeling stuck and can't get yourself motivated to enjoy some self-care*, try *These Three Things.*

1. **Countdown**—Whether you start at 10 or 3, countdown to GO! It may be a barely audible whisper. You may shout it at the top of your lungs. Setting the immediate goal that "I'm going to get up at GO" does the trick when you are lacking motivation.
2. **Play a Pump-Up Song**—Put on a song that you know will inspire you, that will get your foot tapping and your hips shaking or that you can sing along to will fill you with energy. Remember Newton's Law? An object in motion stays in motion. Once you're moving it is easier to keep moving and start that healthy activity.
3. **Repeat your WHY**—Why are you doing this? Why is this moment of self-care important? "I need to stay healthy so that I can take care of my mom." Or "I need to do this so that my blood pressure stays down." Or "I'm doing this for my own sanity." Whatever your WHY, say it out loud.

Multiple times. As many times as you need to hear it. This way you're thinking it, saying it, and hearing it. It may feel uncomfortable at first, but it will help motivate you to get moving.

1. Support groups are incredible resources to learn, have someone to talk with and help you to not feel so alone. You can find support groups in your area online or through your local office on aging.
2. Follow up with your own medical appointments. It is easy to let those slide and before you know it your health is suffering.
3. Be aware of your alcohol intake. Research shows a risk of increased alcohol intake and binge drinking among dementia caregivers. It might take away the edge for a minute, but it is not a long-term solution. In fact, it may lead to more problems and stress [6].
4. Seeking professional support through counseling is very healthy. There are so many emotions that occur when caregiving and none of them are wrong. Two emotions that many caregivers often experience that must be addressed are guilt and anger. It is important to not turn them inward and bury them. Counseling is not a sign of weakness. It is a sign of great strength.
5. Going away for a weekend or longer might be the break that you need. Leaving the person you are caring for with a trusted family member or hiring a professional caregiver is an option. This would give you the opportunity to decompress and reboot your energy.

Whenever you get the chance or whatever the time frame is, it is imperative for you to take time for you. There is no substitute for self-care. And there is no substitute for you.

References

1. Alzheimer's Association. 2023 Alzheimer's disease facts and figures. Alzheimers Dement. 2023;19(4):1598–695. https://doi.org/10.1002/alz.13016.
2. Hellis E, Mukaetova-Ladinska EB. Informal caregiving and Alzheimer's disease: the psychological effect. Medicina. 2023;59(1):48. https://doi.org/10.3390/medicina59010048.
3. NIH: National Institute of Mental Health. Caring for your mental health. 2024. https://www.nimh.nih.gov/health/topics/caring-for-your-mental-health#:~:text=When%20it%20comes%20to%20your,can%20have%20a%20big%20impact.
4. AARP. Daily acts of self-care easing caregiver stress. 2021. https://www.aarp.org/caregiving/life-balance/info-2021/easy-daily-self-care.html.
5. Carney DR, Cuddy AJC, Yap AJ. Power posing: brief nonverbal displays affect neuroendocrine levels and risk tolerance. Psychological Science. 2010;21(10):1363–8. https://doi.org/10.1177/0956797610383437.
6. Secinti E, Wei W, Kent EE, Demark-Wahnefried W, Lewson AB, Mosher CE. Examining health behaviors of chronic disease caregivers in the U.S. American Journal of Preventive Medicine. 2022;62(3):e145–58. https://doi.org/10.1016/j.amepre.2021.07.004.

Chapter 9
Promoting Brain Health

Changes to the brain can start to develop 20 years before the first symptoms of dementia become apparent [1]. Research tells us that there are things that we can do to maintain and improve the health of our brain; therefore, potentially delaying the onset of dementia. There are several risk factors that we can't change such as genes, age, and gender, but there are many that are modifiable. Adopting a healthy lifestyle at any point in our lives can potentially add years to our brain's health [2].

According to a 2020 study reported in Neuroscience News, 40% of dementias can be prevented [3] by addressing *These Three Things*:

1. **Increase**

    (a) Physical Activity—There are conflicting reports on the type, duration, and frequency of physical activity needed for dementia prevention; however, it is unanimous that any type of physical activity is a benefit. Often people have the misconception that physical activity means 60 min of high-intensity, sweat producing, fast-paced movement every day. When in fact, physical activity is simply increasing the amount of movement you do every day with the goal of progressing to consistent aerobic exercise. Increase your daily steps. Take the steps instead of the elevator. Enjoy a random dance party in your family room. Join a sports league—pickleball, kickball, or golf. Please consult your medical provider before starting any physical activity.

    (b) Healthy Food Choices

    Research shows that diets focused on vegetables, fruits, whole grains, nut, and fish promote brain health. These foods improve our cardiovascular health, reduce inflammation, and nourish the brain protecting it from oxidative stress. A healthy diet limits sugar, processed food, fried food, red meat, and saturated fats. Although they may be an easy source of energy, they contribute to health conditions that are negatively linked to dementia. They do not provide our bodies with valued nutrients.

L. Jenkins et al., *These Three Things*,
https://doi.org/10.1007/978-3-031-69394-6_9

A healthy eating style is not only about the types of food it is also about the portions. It is about setting yourself up to maintain healthy food habits. Dietitians are great resources to help learn about and develop these healthy food habits [1, 4, 5].

(c) Socialization—More and more research studies are showing that strong social ties are crucial to your brain health. Interacting with others stimulates your brain by strengthening your brain networks and promoting cell repair. In a time when technology is overtaking our interactions with others, it is imperative to maintain those in-person connections [6]. Schedule a coffee date with a friend. Meet a friend for a walk in the park. Stop and chat with your neighbor. Join a book or other social club.

(d) Brain Activity—People who regularly challenge their mind build a cognitive reserve. Mental exercises may increase the connections between brain cells and promote new networks between cells. Mentally active people can afford to lose a few brain cells due to that reserve hence delaying the onset of dementia. There is no prescription for the type of brain activity that is best. The key is to keep your brain active and challenged doing what is best for you [7, 8]. Work on a crossword puzzle. Learn a new language. Write your grocery list using your non-dominant hand. Play a game on your phone or computer. Drive home a different route.

2. **Decrease**

(a) Smoking—It is known that smoking increases the risk of vascular problems including strokes and brain bleeds contributing to dementia. Toxins from nicotine cause inflammation and stress to brain cells which are both linked to the onset of dementia. While smoking cessation is ideal, any reduction is a benefit [9].

(b) Alcohol—"Over a long period of time people who drink heavily can have reduced volume of the brain's white matter which helps to transmit messages throughout the brain." [10] Long-term heavy consumption may result in a lack of vitamin thiamine-B1. This can cause a short-term memory disorder called Korsakoff's Syndrome. Research is mixed on the effects of moderate alcohol consumption [11].

(c) Obesity—Excess body fat increases inflammation which contributes to the buildup of damaging proteins in the brain. Surplus weight around your middle and elevated BMIs have been linked to an increased risk for developing dementia [12, 13].

(d) Stress—Stress effects the immune system. As we age, the ability of the immune system to fight off infection decreases while allowing chronic low-grade inflammation to increase [14]. A key hormone released during stress, cortisol, has been linked to problems with memory [15, 16]. Managing stress plays an important role in decreasing our risk for dementia. Refer to the chapter on self-care for tips for managing stress.

3. **Avoid**

(a) Traumatic Brain Injury (TBI)/Head Trauma—One of the most feared long-term consequences of TBI is dementia. This type of injury is most frequently association with frontal-temporal lobe dementia. Practicing safe driving practices such as wearing your seatbelt, wearing helmets when playing sports or riding a motorcycle and avoiding contact sports are ways to potentially avoid head trauma [17, 18].

(b) Environmental factors—The impact of the environment on dementia has become a large focus of current research. Air pollution is the most implicated environmental factor contributing to dementia. It is not only the type of pollutant, but the duration of exposure. Practicing safety measures can reduce the exposure to dangerous particles [19]. Check the air quality forecast in your area. On days when the quality is poor, limit your time outside. Avoid exercising in high traffic areas. Consistently change the air filters in your furnace.

By focusing on overall health through increasing, decreasing, and avoiding the things above, you can actively take steps to reduce your dementia risk. Lifestyle changes can be hard. Every single step that you take forward adds to your brain's health moving you one step farther away from a dementia diagnosis.

References

1. Alzheimer's Association. 2023 Alzheimer's disease facts and figures. Alzheimers Dementia. 2023;19(4):1598–695. https://doi.org/10.1002/alz.13016.
2. Alzheimer's Association. 10 healthy habits for your brain. 2024. https://www.alz.org/help-support/brain_health/10-healthy-habits-for-your-brain.
3. Neuroscience News. 40% of dementia cases could be prevented or delayed by targeting 12 risk factors throughout life. 2020. https://neurosciencenews.com/dementia-prevention-life-16748/.
4. NIH: National Institute of Mental Health. What do we know about diet and the prevention of Alzheimer's. https://www.nia.nih.gov/health/alzheimers-and-dementia/what-do-we-know-about-diet-and-prevention-alzheimers-disease.
5. Harvard T.H. Chan School of Public Health. Diet review: the MIND diet. 2023. https://www.hsph.harvard.edu/nutritionsource/healthy-weight/diet-reviews/mind-diet/#:~:text=Researchers%20found%20a%2053%25%20lower,with%20the%20lowest%20MIND%20scores.
6. Solan M. Protecting yourself from Alzheimer's. 2023. https://www.health.harvard.edu/mind-and-mood/protecting-yourself-from-alzheimers#:~:text=Stimulation.,doing%20puzzles%2C%20and%20playing%20games.
7. Harvard Health Publishing: Harvard Medical School. 12 ways to keep your brain young. 2022. https://www.health.harvard.edu/mind-and-mood/12-ways-to-keep-your-brain-young.
8. Wilson RS, Wang T, Yu L, Grodstein F, Bennett DA, Boyle PA. Cognitive activity and onset age of incident alzheimer disease dementia. Neurology. 2021;97(9):e922–9. https://doi.org/10.1212/wnl.0000000000012388.
9. Alzheimer's Society. Smoking and the risk of dementia. 2023. https://www.alzheimers.org.uk/about-dementia/managing-the-risk-of-dementia/reduce-your-risk-of-dementia/smoking.

10. Alzheimer's Society. Alcohol and the risk of dementia. 2023. https://www.alzheimers.org.uk/about-dementia/managing-the-risk-of-dementia/reduce-your-risk-of-dementia/alcohol.
11. Jeonm KH, Han K, Jeong S, et al. Changes in alcohol consumption and risk of dementia in a nationwide cohort in South Korea. JAMA Netw Open. 2023;6(2):e2254771. https://doi.org/10.1001/jamanetworkopen.2022.54771.
12. Flores-Cordero JA, Pérez-Pérez A, Jiménez-Cortegana C, Alba G, Flores-Barragán A, Sánchez-Margalet V. Obesity as a risk factor for dementia and Alzheimer's disease: the role of leptin. Int J Mol Sci. 2022;23(9):5202. https://doi.org/10.3390/ijms23095202.
13. Salas-Venegas V, Flores-Torres RP, Rodríguez-Cortés YM, Rodríguez-Retana D, Ramírez-Carreto RJ, Concepción-Carrillo LE, Pérez-Flores LJ, Alarcón-Aguilar A, López-Díazguerrero NE, Gómez-González B, Chavarría A, Konigsberg M. The obese brain: mechanisms of systemic and local inflammation, and interventions to reverse the cognitive deficit. Front Integr Neurosci. 2022;16:798995. https://doi.org/10.3389/fnint.2022.798995.
14. Weyand CM, Goronzy JJ. Aging of the immune system. Mechanisms and therapeutic targets. Ann Am Thorac Soc. 2016;13 Suppl 5(Suppl 5):S422–8. https://doi.org/10.1513/AnnalsATS.201602-095AW.
15. Wallensten J, Ljunggren G, Nager A, et al. Stress, depression, and risk of dementia—a cohort study in the total population between 18 and 65 years old in Region Stockholm. Alz Res Therapy. 2023;15:161. https://doi.org/10.1186/s13195-023-01308-4.
16. Harvard Health Publishing. Protect your brain from stress. 2021. https://www.health.harvard.edu/mind-and-mood/protect-your-brain-from-stress.
17. Alzheimer's Association. Traumatic Brain Injury (TBI). 2024. https://www.alz.org/alzheimers-dementia/what-is-dementia/related_conditions/traumatic-brain-injury.
18. Center for Disease Control and Prevention. Traumatic Brain Injury & Concussion (TBI): prevention. 2021. https://www.cdc.gov/traumaticbraininjury/prevention.html.
19. Knobel P, Litke R, Mobbs CV. Biological age and environmental risk factors for dementia and stroke: Molecular mechanisms. Front Aging Neurosci. 2022;14:1042488. https://doi.org/10.3389/fnagi.2022.1042488.

Glossary

Activities of daily living Activities related to personal care. They include bathing or showering, dressing, getting in and out of bed or a chair, walking, using the toilet, and eating [1].

Aggression The forceful or overly assertive pursuit of one's aims and interests [2].

Anger A strong feeling of annoyance, displeasure, or hostility [3].

Anxiety A feeling of worry, nervousness, or unease, typically about an imminent event or something with an uncertain outcome [4].

Basic needs Making sure that the person has the essentials that are required for optimal functioning. The essentials are food, water, comfort (temperature, clothing), has gone to the bathroom, and has some sort of activity to keep them occupied.

Communication The imparting or exchanging of information or news [5].

Creativity The use of your imagination, the ability to generate or recognize ideas, alternatives, or possibilities [6].

Critical thinking The objective analysis and evaluation of an issue in order to form a judgment [7].

Daylight savings time In countries in the Northern Hemisphere, clocks are usually set ahead 1 h in late March or in April and are set back 1 h in late September or in October [8].

Delirium A disturbed state of mind or consciousness, an acute, transient condition associated with intoxication, fever, and certain other physical disorders characterized by symptoms such as confusion, disorientation, agitation, and hallucinations [9].

Delusions A false belief or judgment about external reality, held despite incontrovertible evidence to the contrary, occurring especially in mental conditions [10].

Dementia A general term for loss of memory, language, problem-solving, and other thinking abilities that are severe enough to interfere with daily life. It is not a specific disease [11].

Distraction A thing that prevents someone from giving full attention to something else [12].

Elopement A person with cognitive impairment wanders away or leaves an area without supervision or authorization and presents a safety threat to the (person) and/or others [13].

Emergency Response System (ERS) Electronic devices which when triggered initiate a call for help.

Enter their reality Accepting the person's current version of reality and merging with them in that moment. For example, if you are helping them get ready for a doctor's appointment and they think that they are getting ready to go to school, act as if they are getting ready to go to school. If it is June and they think it is October, talk about the fall season.

Essential oils A form of alternative medicine that employs plants extracts to support health and wellbeing. Changes in a person's sense of smell will not impact the effectiveness of essential oils [14].

Exit seeking behaviors Attempting to leave the room or home as a means of looking to fulfill a need or escape a situation.

Fall risk Any item of event that would lead to an unintended descent to the floor. For example, throw rugs, unsteady gait, improper footwear.

Fidget box A container that holds small items or objects that the person can sort or play with to distract or hold their attention.

Five words or less A concept to use no more than five words when giving direction or communicating. "Come with me." "Let's go this way." "It's time for dinner."

Flexibility The willingness to change or compromise, having patience [15].

Hallucinations A false perception of objects or events involving your senses: sights, sounds, touch, and taste. They seem real but they are not [16].

Hoarding Persistent difficulty getting rid of or parting with possessions due to a perceived need to save the item [17].

Hyperorality (Hyper Oral) Exploring the world through their mouth. Overeat, eat things that aren't food or have mouth-centered compulsive behaviors [18].

Incontinence Lack of ability to control the bladder and bowels [19].

Mindfulness A mental state achieved by focusing one's awareness on the present moment, while calmly acknowledging and accepting one's feelings, thoughts, and bodily sensations, used as a therapeutic technique [20].

Mirror image Perform a task in front of or in the sight of the person with the goal of them copying your actions.

Nonverbal communication The act of conveying information without the use of words. Nonverbal communication occurs through facial expressions, gestures, body language, tone of voice, and other physical indications of mood and attitude [21].

Over stimulation Multiple things happening at once that overwhelm the senses causing the brain to shut down. For example: excess noise, too much activity, bright or flashing lights.

Paranoia A state of mind in which the individual has a strong belief that he/she is persecuted by others and therefore displays behaviors marked by suspiciousness [22].

Pocketing food The action of chewing your food and pushing it into your cheeks or teeth without the act of swallowing it.

Quality of life The standard of health, comfort, and happiness as experienced by the person, in the terms that matters to the person.

Redirection To change the focus from one task to another.

Routine The normal order and way in which you regularly do things [23].

Shadowing When a person with dementia constantly follows their caregiver around.

Sleep hygiene Practicing daily routines that support your body's natural ability to fall asleep, reach deep sleep, and stay asleep throughout the night [24].

Spaced retrieval The act of writing down the answer to a repeatedly asked question or important information in order to help the person with dementia remember [25, 26]. Tips for using spaced retrieval: Utilize five words or less. Use a dark print on a solid light-colored piece of paper. Print with big letters. Only provide the information that is being asked.

Stimulation The act of encouraging of something so that it develops or becomes more active, the act of making someone interested and excited about something by engaging their mind or physical senses [27].

Sundowning A term used for changes in behavior that occur in the evening around dusk [28].

Therapeutic truths A communication strategy where you jump into the person's reality with a fib to calm or redirect their anxiety, fear, or confusion. Some people struggle with the idea of fibbing, but you are speaking their truth in the moment and the outcome is in their best interest.

Tinker box A container filled with items that stimulate the senses to occupy or distract the person. The items should be personalized to the interests of the person. For example: pictures, plastic silverware, a deck of cards, buttons, fidget spinner, acorns.

Toileting schedule Taking the person to or prompting them to use the bathroom at predetermined times throughout the day. For example, every 2 hours while awake.

Tracking behaviors Writing down the date, time, and mood surrounding an event or behavior over several hours or days in order to identify a possible trigger or trend.

Triangulate When two people who are involved in a conflict attempt to involve a third party [29].

Triggers Experiencing a negative or undesirable emotional or behavioral reaction in response to a current situation that causes distress. For example: over stimulation triggering agitated or irritable behavior.

Urinary Tract Infection (UTI) Infection in any part of the urinary system. Also referred to as a bladder infection. This can occur more often in older adults with incontinence, dehydration, poor personal hygiene, sitting in wet incontinence products. Serious health issues can result if left untreated [30].

Validate Recognize or affirm the validity or worth of a person or their feelings or opinions: cause a person to feel valued or worthwhile [32].

Word salad A confused or unintelligible mixture of seemingly words or phrases [31].

References

1. Oxford English Dictionary. Activities of daily living. In: oed.com dictionary. https://www.oed.com/search/dictionary/?scope=Entries&q=activities+of+daily+living. Accessed 1 Apr 2024.
2. Oxford English Dictionary. Aggression. In: oed.com dictionary. https://www.oed.com/search/dictionary/?scope=Entries&q=aggression. Accessed 1 Apr 2024.
3. Oxford English Dictionary. Anger. In: oed.com dictionary. https://www.oed.com/search/dictionary/?scope=Entries&q=anger. Accessed 1 Apr 2024.
4. Oxford English Dictionary. Anxiety. In: oed.com dictionary. https://www.oed.com/search/dictionary/?scope=Entries&q=anxiety. Accessed 1 Apr 2024.
5. Oxford English Dictionary. Communication. In: oed.com dictionary. https://www.oed.com/search/dictionary/?scope=Entries&q=communication. Accessed 1 Apr 2024.
6. Oxford English Dictionary. Creativity. In: oed.com dictionary. https://www.oed.com/search/dictionary/?scope=Entries&q=creativity. Accessed 1 Apr 2024.
7. Oxford English Dictionary. Critical thinking. In: oed.com dictionary. https://www.oed.com/search/dictionary/?scope=Entries&q=critical+thinking. Accessed 1 Apr 2024.
8. Betts JD. Daylight saving time. Encyclopedia Britannica; 2023. https://www.britannica.com/topic/Daylight-Saving-Time
9. Oxford English Dictionary. Delirium. In: oed.com dictionary. https://www.oed.com/search/dictionary/?scope=Entries&q=delirium+. Accessed 1 Apr 2024.
10. Oxford English Dictionary. Delirium. In: oed.com dictionary. https://www.oed.com/search/dictionary/?scope=Entries&q=delusions+. Accessed 1 Apr 2024.
11. Alzheimer's and Dementia. Alzheimer's Association; 2024. https://www.alz.org/alzheimer_s_dementia.
12. Oxford English Dictionary. Distraction. In: oed.com dictionary. https://www.oed.com/search/dictionary/?scope=Entries&q=distraction. Accessed 1 Apr 2024.
13. PACE Quality monitoring & reporting guidance. Center of Medicare Services; 2021. www.cms.gov/files/document/pacequalitymonitoringandreportingguidancemarch2021.pdf.
14. West H. What are essential oils, and do they work? Healthline Magazine. 2019. https://www.healthline.com/nutrition/what-are-essential-oils.
15. Oxford Learners Dictionary. Flexibility. In: oxfordlearnersdictionaries.com dictionary. https://www.oxfordlearnersdictionaries.com/us/definition/english/flexibility?q=flexibility. Accessed 1 Apr 2024.
16. Hallucinations. Cleveland Clinic Health Library; 2022. https://my.clevelandclinic.org/health/symptoms/23350-hallucinations.

17. What is hoarding disorder? American Psychiatric Association; 2021. https://www.psychiatry. org/patients-families/hoarding-disorder/what-is-hoarding-disorder.

18. Hernandez A. Hyperorality. What is it, causes, treatment and more, Osmosis from Elsevier; 2024. https://www.osmosis.org/answers/hyperorality.

19. Oxford English Dictionary. Incontinence. In: oed.com dictionary. https://www.oed.com/ search/dictionary/?scope=Entries&q=incontinence. Accessed 1 Apr 2024.

20. Oxford English Dictionary. Mindfulness. In: oed.com dictionary. https://www.oed.com/ search/dictionary/?scope=Entries&q=mindfulness. Accessed 1 Apr 2024.

21. APA Dictionary of Psychology. Nonverbal communication. In: apa.org dictionary. https://dictionary.apa.org/nonverbal-communication. Accessed 1 Apr 2024.

22. Oxford English Dictionary. Paranoia. In: oed.com dictionary. https://www.oed.com/search/dictionary/?scope=Entries&q=paranoia. Accessed 1 Apr 2024.

23. Oxford English Dictionary. Routine. In: oed.com dictionary. https://www.oed.com/search/dictionary/?scope=Entries&q=routine&tl=true. Accessed 1 Apr 2024.

24. Pugle M. What is Sleep Hygiene: good sleeping habits are foundational to your health. Very Well Health; 2022. https://www.verywellhealth.com/ sleep-hygiene-definition-types-techniques-efficacy-6749577.

25. Carpenter SK, Pan SC, Butler AC. The science of effective learning with spacing and retrieval practice. Nat Rev. Psychol. 2022;1:496–511. https://doi.org/10.1038/s44159-022-00089-1.

26. Small JA, Cochrane D. Spaced retrieval and episodic memory training in Alzheimer's disease. Clin Interv Aging. 2020;15:519–36. https://doi.org/10.2147/CIA.S242113.

27. Oxford English Dictionary. Stimulation. In: oed.com dictionary. https://www.oed.com/search/dictionary/?scope=Entries&q=stimulation. Accessed 1 Apr 2024.

28. Sundowning (Changes in Behaviours at Dusk). 2023. https://www.dementiauk.org/ information-and-support/health-advice/sundowning/

29. Guha A. Understanding Triangulation: what to do when someone draws you into a personal conflict. Psychology Today. 2021. https://www.psychologytoday/us/ blog-prisons-and-pathos/202110/understanding:triangulation.

30. Diseases and conditions: UTI. Mayo Clinic; 2022. https://www.mayoclinic.org/ diseases-conditions/urinary-tract-infection/symptoms-causes/syc-20353447.

31. Oxford English Dictionary. Word salad. In: oed.com dictionary. https://www.oed.com/search/dictionary/?scope=Entries&q=word+salad. Accessed 1 Apr 2024.

32. Oxford English Dictionary. Validate. In: oed.com dictionary. https://www.oed.com/search/dictionary/?scope=Entries&q=validate. Accessed 1 Apr 2024.

Index

Endoscopic Third Ventriculostomy

Roberto Alexandre Dezena

Endoscopic Third Ventriculostomy

Classic Concepts and a
State-of-the-Art Guide

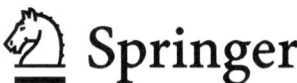 Springer

Roberto Alexandre Dezena, MD, PhD
Division of Neurosurgery
Federal University of Triângulo Mineiro
Uberaba, Minas Gerais, Brazil

ISBN 978-3-030-28656-9   ISBN 978-3-030-28657-6   (eBook)
https://doi.org/10.1007/978-3-030-28657-6

This Springer imprint is published by the registered company Springer Nature Switzerland AG
The registered company address is: Gewerbestrasse 11, 6330 Cham, Switzerland

To my dear and beloved wife, Fabiana, my source of peace and inspiration

Foreword

Since the beginning of the use of neuroendoscopy, the treatment of hydrocephalus has been the main objective. For more than a hundred years, the technical and therapeutic efforts have been aimed at improving the technique and its results. Also, education through numerous congresses, symposia, and workshops around the world during the last 20 years has strengthened and consolidated the procedure, as well as a new way of understanding the physiopathology of the circulation of the cerebrospinal fluid. Many of the dogmas of the past have fallen, opening the way to new concepts of treatment. It is strictly necessary that this knowledge encompasses not only the neurosurgeons but also to its clinical environment, i.e., to its anesthesiology team of intensive care of adult and pediatric patients, internal medicine, and neurology. The ISGNE - International Study Group of Neuroendoscopy, transformed into IFNE - International Federation of Neuroendoscopy, was founded in 2001 so that the experience of the great Masters was transmitted and applied by all of us. No doubt at the beginning of the new millennium, minimal invasion neurosurgery will be more consolidated. This book will be one step further in that theoretical effort to bring by hand the development of new instruments capable of improving the technical limitations of the procedure.

Montevideo, Uruguay   Alvaro Cordoba, MD, FMUW

Preface

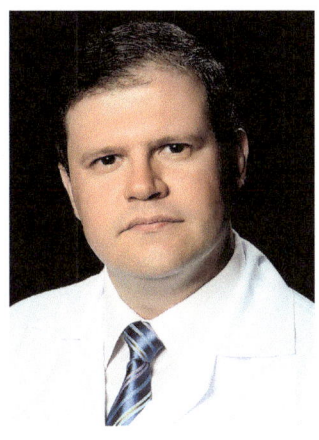

The endoscopic third ventriculostomy is the most performed neuroendoscopic procedure in the world, and for this reason, it is widely studied. Its in-depth knowledge is extremely important for all who propose to treat hydrocephalus patients by neuroendoscopy. New knowledge is constantly emerging, especially in the indications of the technique in childhood hydrocephalus. The aim of this book is to concentrate and disseminate such knowledge in a practical and direct way. By no means is it a book directed to experts in the subject, but to those who are taking the first steps in neuroendoscopy. The work is divided into two parts. Part I, in Chaps. 1 and 2, discusses classical concepts, such as historical aspects of the evolution of the treatment of hydrocephalus and anatomical and physiological aspects of the ventricular system. Such concepts are extremely important because they are the basis for understanding the indications. In Part II, current knowledge about the neuroendoscopic technique, essential for the success of the procedures, is exposed. Chapters 3 and 4 discuss endoscopic ventricular anatomy and general aspects of the neuroendoscopic technique, useful for any endoscopic neurosurgery. Endoscopic third ventriculostomy, especially in terms of indication and its association with the coagulation of the choroid plexus, which is widely used in children, still controversial, and endoscopic third ventriculostomy surgical technique are thoroughly discussed in Chaps. 5 and 6, respectively. Online videos illustrate these chapters.

Chapter 7 sets out new way of treating obstructive hydrocephalus by neuroendoscopy. Far from being the final word on the subject, we hope that this humble and unpretentious work can be useful for the benefit of patients all over the world.

Uberaba, Minas Gerais, Brazil   Roberto Alexandre Dezena, MD, PhD

Contents

Part I
Classic Concepts

Chapter 1
Historical Aspects of Hydrocephalus and Its Treatments

1.1 Development of the Concept of Hydrocephalus

1.1.1 Anatomical and Physiological Bases

The word hydrocephalus is derived from the Greek words "head" and "water." Hippocrates (ca. 460 BC ca. 370 BC) mentions this disease, which he imagined as intracranial fluids concentrated outside the brain. Hippocrates is also credited for the first ventricular puncture [1]. However, it is unlikely that children with increased cephalic volume went unnoticed by Hippocrates' ancestors. Around the time of Christ, the focus of civilization moved on from Greece to Rome. At this time, Claudius Galen (ca. 129 ca. 217), with his vast knowledge of anatomy, recognized the importance of the choroid plexus and ventricular cavities and believed that these were the source of the animal spirit (*pneumapsychikon*). He conceived the idea that the fluid that the brain was immersed in was a dynamic, moving fluid absorbed by the cribriform plate and the pituitary body. His description of hydrocephalus resembled that of Hippocrates, in that he did not relate the phenomenon to ventricular dilatation [2]. Galen's knowledge prevailed throughout the Dark Ages, since at that time dissections of corpses were not permitted. It was only in the late Middle Ages that dissection was occasionally permitted in some universities, such as Paris (1150), Bologna (1158), Oxford (1167), Montpellier (1181), and Padua (1222) [3]. New anatomical concepts emerged when dissection became more commonplace, which was possible with the advent of the Renaissance. Without a doubt, his greatest representative was Leonardo da Vinci (1452–1519), who did an exceptional work by injecting solidifying substances into the ventricular cavity, removing the brain tissue, and thus building the first model of the ventricular system [4]. Another great representative of the period was Andreas Vesalius (1514–1564), who studied at the University of Padua, where he based his best-known studies. His greatest work, *De humani corporis fabrica libri septem* or *De humani corporis fabrica*, or simply *Fabrica*, dated 1543, is considered by many authors the greatest book in the history

© Springer Nature Switzerland AG 2020   3
R. A. Dezena, *Endoscopic Third Ventriculostomy*,
https://doi.org/10.1007/978-3-030-28657-6_1

of science, which definitively established the connection between human anatomy and physiology. Vesalius described a child with hydrocephalus, recognized the accumulation of fluid inside the ventricular system, and suspected that this excessive fluid could cause cerebral destruction that accompanies hydrocephalus [5]. If the Renaissance established the anatomical bases, the seventeenth century established the physiological bases of medicine. William Harvey (1578–1657) described the circulation of blood, and Thomas Bartholin (1616–1680) is credited with the discovery of the lymphatic system. Thomas Willis (1621–1675), who made important descriptions regarding cerebral circulation, hypothesized that the cerebrospinal fluid (CSF) was secreted in the choroid plexus and drained into the venous system [6]. Despite advances in the understanding of body fluids, since ancient times there was a great deal of discussion as to whether the fluid inside the ventricular cavity was gaseous or liquid. The definition of its true liquid nature would come only in 1764 with Domenico Felice Antonio Cotugno (1736–1822), who recognized it as an aqueous medium and not a vapor, as Galen believed, and that it was present in the ventricles. In the seventeenth and eighteenth centuries, beautiful illustrations of the hydrocephalus phenomenon appeared (Figs. 1.1 and 1.2 [7, 8]). In the eighteenth

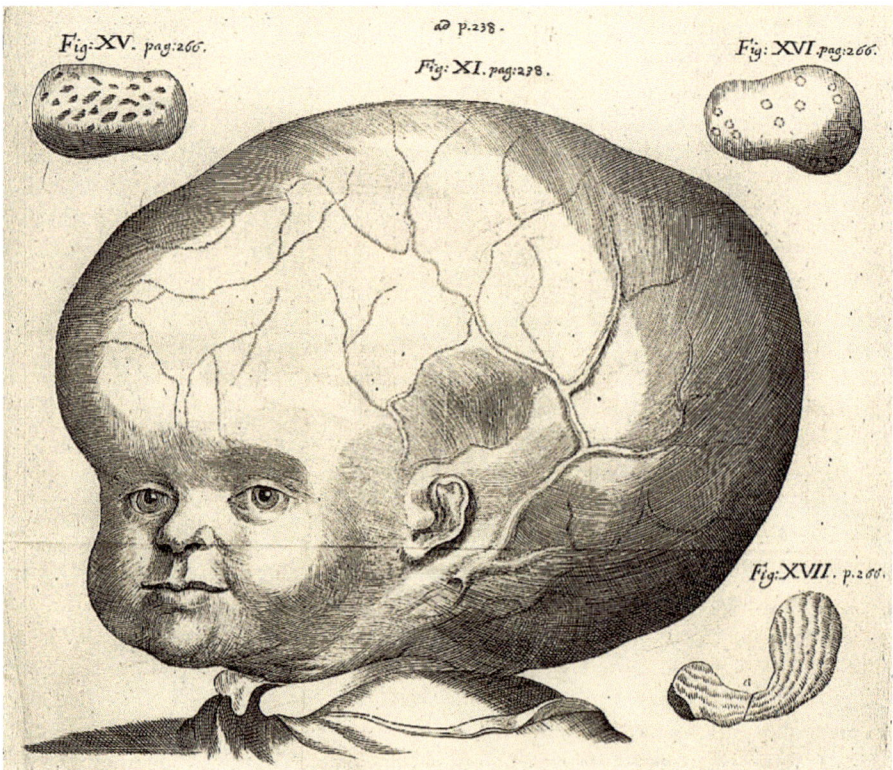

Fig. 1.1 Beautiful illustration of a child with hydrocephalus, of 1696, with evident venous engorgement of the scalp. (Reprinted from Schroeck [7])

Fig. 1.2 Curious illustration of a child with hydrocephalus, 1702, holding part of a placenta. (Reprinted from Ruysch [8])

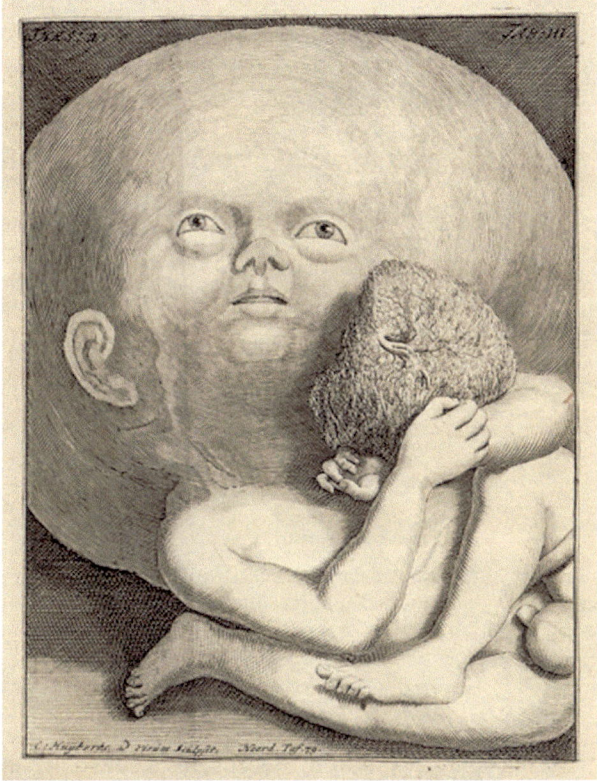

century, the knowledge about hydrocephalus advanced under the aegis of scientific experiments and careful clinical observations. Franz de le Boë (1614–1672), or *Franciscus Sylvius*, in its Latinized form, described the cerebral aqueduct, Antonio Pacchioni (1665–1726) described the dura mater and subarachnoid granulations [9] (Fig. 1.3), and Alexander Monro secundus (1733–1817) described the interventricular foramina. Albrecht von Haller (1708–1777), creator of experimental physiology, described the pathophysiology of hydrocephalus from experiments on animals. Robert Whytt (1714–1766) gave the first description of the clinical aspects of hydrocephalus and the consequences of intracranial hypertension. Giovanni Battista Morgagni (1682–1771), a pioneer of anatomical-clinical correlation from autopsies, provided a detailed description of the pathology of hydrocephalus, in his masterpiece *De Sedibus* in 1761 [10] (Fig. 1.4). Jean Cruveilhier (1791–1874) made important contributions in his studies involving the nervous system, including the pathophysiology of hydrocephalus [11] (Fig. 1.5). François Jean Magendie (1783–1855) and Hubert von Luschka (1820–1875) described the fourth ventricular outflow tracts. Finally, the monumental work of Axel Key (1832–1901) and Magnus Gustaf Retzius (1842–1919) from 1876 described in detail the subarachnoid space, establishing the dynamics of CSF circulation [2].

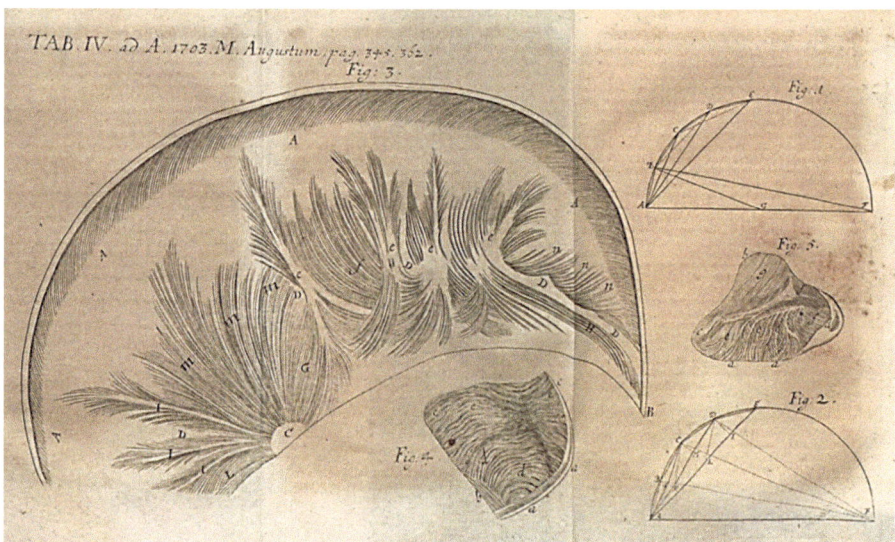

Fig. 1.3 Illustration of the dura mater with detailed description, which allowed the discovery of arachnoid granulations. (Reprinted from Pacchioni [9])

1.1.2   Attempts of Treatment

No clinical treatment of hydrocephalus resulted in a definitive solution to the problem. Osmotic agents such as Mannitol and Glycerol as well as Acetazolamide, which reduce CSF production, are used only for transient relief of intracranial hypertension associated with hydrocephalus. By the end of the nineteenth century, the anatomical, physiological, and clinical bases of hydrocephalus were established. The need to solve the problem had become clear. As such, hydrocephalus was a potentially fatal and inexorably progressive disease. Before the advent of some form of surgical treatment, almost nothing could be done to stop its progression. Numerous forms of treatment began with William Williams Keen Jr. (1837–1932) (Fig. 1.6), in 1888, who established continuous external ventricular drainage. Heinrich Irenaeus Quincke (1842–1922), in 1891, proposed using intermittent lumbar punctures. Despite the pioneering work of Keen and Quincke, such attempts at treatment failed to achieve more than a temporary relief from the pathological process. At this stage, Walter Edward Dandy (1886–1946) began his studies whose results would forever change the management of hydrocephalus. In a series of experiments between 1913 and 1929, he established the true dynamic pathology of hydrocephalus and summed up the principles for its causal treatment based on the knowledge he acquired. Using X-rays, he developed ventriculography in 1918, which offered for the first time the opportunity to visualize and measure the ventricular cavity in patients before and after surgery. Dandy further studied CSF circulation with dyes and classified hydrocephalus as communicating if the dye injected into the ventricles could be recovered in the lumbar subarachnoid space and as obstructive if it could not. Between 1918

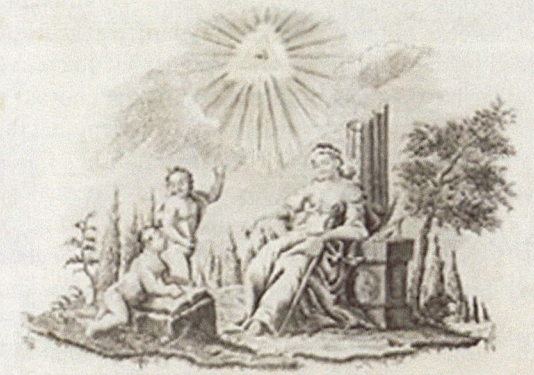

JO. BAPTISTÆ
MORGAGNI
P. P. P. P.
DE SEDIBUS, ET CAUSIS
MORBORUM
PER ANATOMEN INDAGATIS
LIBRI QUINQUE.

DISSECTIONES, ET ANIMADVERSIONES, NUNC PRIMUM EDITAS
COMPLECTUNTUR PROPEMODUM INNUMERAS, MEDICIS,
CHIRURGIS, ANATOMICIS PROFUTURAS.

Multiplex præfixus eſt Index rerum, & nominum
accuratiſſimus.

TOMUS PRIMUS
DUOS PRIORES CONTINENS LIBROS.

VENETIIS,
MDCCLXI.
EX TYPOGRAPHIA REMONDINIANA.
SUPERIORUM PERMISSU, AC PRIVILEGIO.

Fig. 1.4 The frontispiece of *De Sedibus*. (Reprinted from Morgagni [10])

Fig. 1.5 Illustration of a 9-month-old child with hydrocephalus resulting from meningitis, from Cruveilhier's book, with more than 200 illustrations by the painter Antoine Chazal (1793–1854). (Reprinted from Cruveilhier [12])

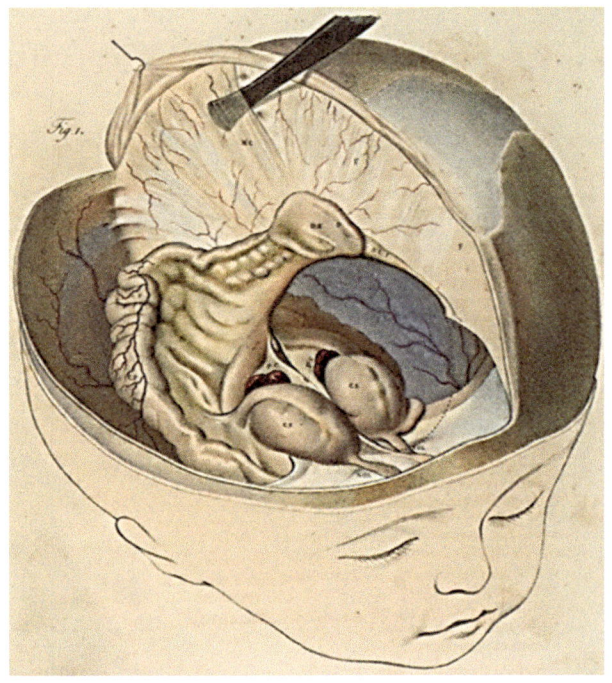

and 1922, Dandy established three principles for the treatment of hydrocephalus, starting with determining the type of hydrocephalus (communicating or obstructive). In obstructive hydrocephalus, ventricular fluid should be drained to the subarachnoid space at the base of the brain, through third ventriculostomy, from where it would be absorbed by natural physiological processes. In communicating hydrocephalus, on the other hand, surgical destruction of the choroid plexus should be performed in order to reduce CSF production to an amount that the malfunctioning absorption system could handle [13, 14]. Having established these principles, various techniques were developed to perform the third ventriculostomy in order to facilitate internal diversion of the cerebrospinal fluid. The first one, described by Dandy himself in 1922, was performed through subfrontal access and section of a healthy optic nerve [15]. The introduction of silicone, a new biocompatible synthetic material, to medicine in 1947, changed the approach to treatment of hydrocephalus from the guidelines established by Dandy. In 1949, Frank Nulsen (1916–1994) and Eugene Spitz (1919–2006) introduced the concept of shunt as a new method of treating hydrocephalus by draining the CSF into the atrium and the peritoneum [16]. In 1955, John Holter (1916–2003) introduced a one-way valve system, which was inspired by the death of his son Casey, due to complications from post-myelomeningocele hydrocephalus [17]. These shunt techniques became benchmarks in the treatment of hydrocephalus, due to the high rate of complications associated with neuroendoscopy, which was taking its first steps. So third ventriculostomy, endoscopic or not, has been ostracized and regarded as an obsolete procedure rarely indicated or rarely used in services at that time [2].

Fig. 1.6 William Williams Keen Jr. (1837–1932), the first brain surgeon in the United States, by American photographer Theodore Christopher Marceau (1859–1922)

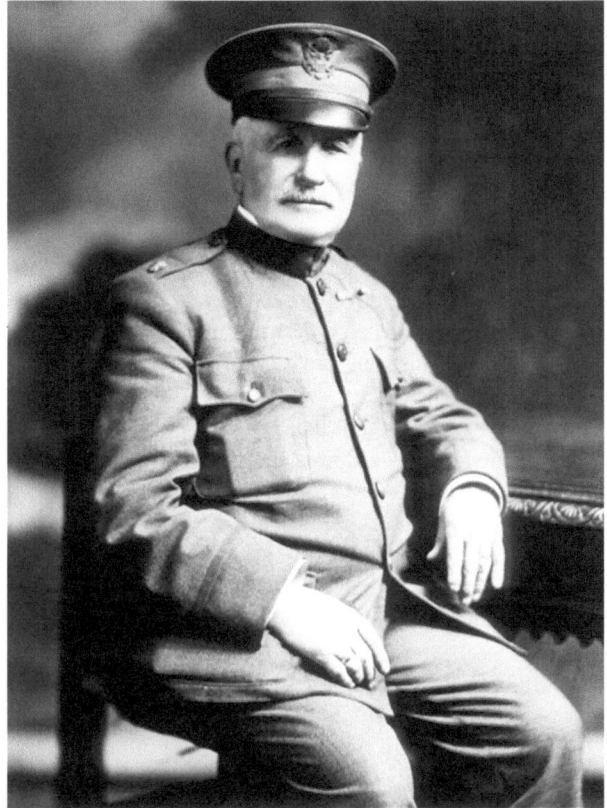

1.2   Treatment of Hydrocephalus Based on the Third Ventricle

Theoretically, the best surgical solution for hydrocephalus would be a procedure that best mimicked nature: a shunt from the subarachnoid space to the superior sagittal sinus with an opening pressure of 70 mmH$_2$O. If a shunt is inserted, it should be made of biocompatible material, and drain from the frontal horn of the lateral ventricle to the superior sagittal sinus. Another alternative would be a ventriculoperitoneal system with anti-siphon mechanism, both with an opening pressure of 70 mmH$_2$O, also made of biocompatible material [18]. Third ventriculostomy, which makes possible the communication of the third ventricle with the subarachnoid space, meets these requirements. Currently, it is performed endoscopically, however, initial experiments used catheters. The basic premise for the success of this procedure is the presence of an operating drainage system, from the arachnoid granulations to the sagittal sinus. This does not occur in cases of communicating hydrocephalus, which can be caused by meningitis or subarachnoid hemorrhage, and in newborns where the system is still poorly developed or where ventricular enlargement itself causes obstruction of the basal cisterns [19]. Therefore, third ventriculostomy would be indicated in obstructive hydrocephalus [20]. The evolution of the technique will be detailed below, which culminated in endoscopic third ventriculostomy (ETV), its peak point.

1.2.1   Third-Fourth Interventriculostomy

The first attempt to clear the cerebral aqueduct has been attributed to Dandy in 1920, with the objective of causal treatment of obstructive hydrocephalus [13]. He argued that it must be difficult to maintain the patency of the reconstruction of an extensive stenosis, but since ventriculography did not differentiate the size of the stenosis, the procedure should be indicated in all cases. The surgical technique consisted of insertion of a catheter through the fourth ventricle, rupturing the adhesion of the aqueduct, and reaching the third ventricle. The catheter was perforated in several places, except the portion in contact with the light of the aqueduct, and anchored to the dura mater of the foramen magnum. The catheter was left in place for 2–3 weeks. After this time, the catheter was removed, and presumably the canal would have been reopened. Dandy treated two patients using this technique, one of whom died of pneumonia 7 weeks after surgery and the other one was in good condition a year later [13] (Fig. 1.7). Leksell, in 1949, stated that aqueductal stenosis, although anatomically small, is a difficult-to-treat neurosurgical problem. In his study, among 71 patients with non-tumoral cerebral aqueduct obstruction, 62 were operated on with disappointing results, both in regard to symptom control and mortality rate. Various surgical techniques were employed: ventriculocisternostomy using the methods proposed by Dandy, Hyndman, and Torkildsen, temporary aqueductal catheterization, insertion of a tube into the aqueduct, and exploratory craniotomy. He affirmed that direct approach to the aqueduct is well tolerated and bears little risk, but the final result depends on the patency of the CSF passage. From then on, he advocated an aqueductal reconstruction technique using a spiral wire tube. Through a small posterior fossa craniotomy, a spiral catheter that is approximately 30 mm long and 3 mm in diameter is led through another catheter into the aqueduct

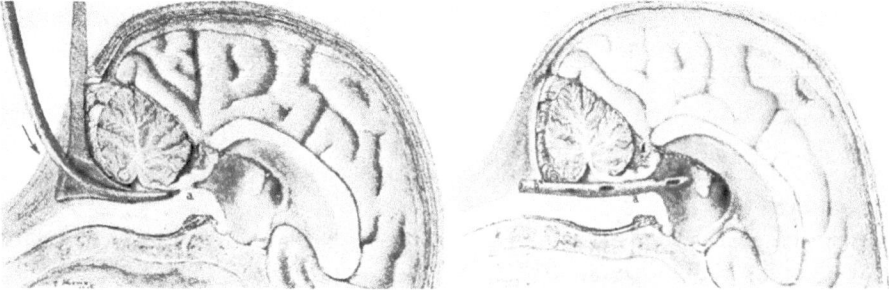

Fig. 1.7 Illustration of the first attempt to treat cerebral aqueduct stenosis. (Reprinted from Dandy [13])

and left there, while the catheter is removed at the end. Of the 13 patients operated on using this technique, 4 died, 2 did not improve, and 7 obtained good results [21]. Elvidge, in 1966, found aqueduct stenosis in 29.5% of the 44 autopsies studied. He found that exploration and catheterization of the aqueduct in children was a dangerous procedure and abandoned it. However, some of these patients reach adolescence or an age when surgery becomes less risky. In his article, he reports the long-term outcomes of ten patients treated by catheterization of the aqueduct with rubber or plastic tubes. The procedure was performed via the fourth ventricle by a posterior fossa craniotomy. Of the 10 patients, one was 7.5 months old, another was 5 weeks old, and all others were over 5 years of age. The tubes were left permanently in eight of the cases, one tube was removed 16 days later, and in one case, none was placed. Two patients died as a result of surgery: one that had no tube placed (due to systemic infection) and one due to epidural hematoma. In addition, of the eight survivors, one patient died 2.5 years later due to non-disease-related reasons, and the other seven achieved long-term survival. He concluded that surgery is feasible and that the carriers can grow into adulthood until the symptoms become harmful and then can be cured by interventriculostomy [22]. During the 1970s, encouraged by the advent of arterial catheterization, Cuatico and Richardson, in 1979, came up with the idea that a catheter could be introduced through the widely open fontanelle of a hydrocephalic patient by percutaneous puncture. Under fluoroscopic control, they introduced an angiography catheter into the lateral ventricle and guided by a simultaneous ventriculography conducted through the aqueduct. The child's symptoms improved immediately, but returned after a few days. They repeated the procedure twice more, using more calibrated catheters, but the good results obtained in the short term did not last more than a few days. They report that the child's parents did not allow a fourth attempt although there were no permanent complications. The child was transferred to another hospital where she underwent a shunt procedure and several subsequent revisions [23] (Fig. 1.8). Avman and Dinçer, in 1980, report the case of a 35-year-old female patient with a history of headaches and who upon examination showed signs of brainstem and intracranial hypertension. A pneumoencephalography revealed obstruction of the cerebral aqueduct. The exploration of the posterior fossa found a venous malformation causing obstruction of the aqueduct. A catheter was passed through the aqueduct and left in place to enable normal CSF circulation. The patient lived normally for another 15 years [24]. Backlund, Grepe, and Lunsford, in 1981, published their experience with cannulating the cerebral aqueduct by stereotactic technique. Prior to surgery, ventriculography was performed by injection of air into the lumbar space that delineated the fourth ventricle and caudal portion of the obstructed aqueduct. A stereotactic head frame is placed, with the patient in the supine position, and frontal trepanation is performed near the midline. Positive intraventricular contrast is injected to delineate the posterior portion of the third ventricle. Superposition of the radiological images (pneumoencephalography and ventriculography) reveals the posterior portion of the third ventricle and the caudal portion of the aqueduct implying stenosis. A Teflon tube measuring 1.5–2.0 cm was inserted to join the two cavities and left there, thus reestablishing interventricular communication. Seven

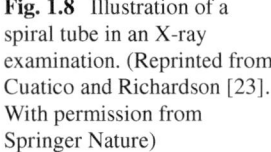

Fig. 1.8 Illustration of a spiral tube in an X-ray examination. (Reprinted from Cuatico and Richardson [23]. With permission from Springer Nature)

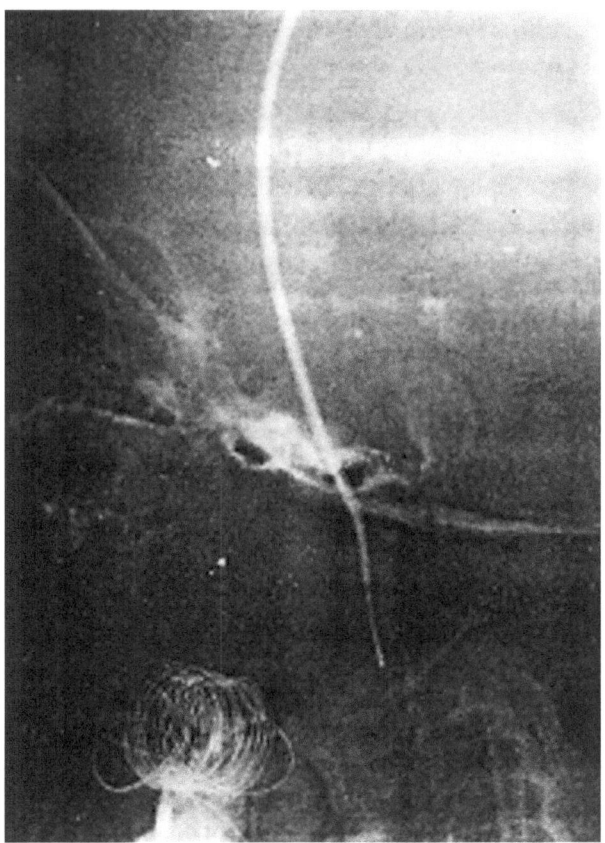

patients underwent 13 procedures. Of these, four patients had prostheses in satisfactory positions, and three had hydrocephalus under good control [25]. Laprat et al., in 1986, have stated that in their experience, the psychological assessment results of children treated with external shunts in childhood are statistically better when evaluated at 5 rather than 10 years of age. They attributed this to the fact that repeated bouts of intracranial hypertension caused by valve dysfunction produce brain lesions early in their lives, which cause inability to live normal lives later. Due to these problems (repeated valve revisions and psychological deterioration) every effort should be made to restore normal routes of CSF circulation early on to achieve compensated hydrocephalus and a normal child without a valve. With this objective, they described a cannulation technique of the aqueduct, via the fourth ventricle, in which a two-pronged catheter is introduced to reestablish the CSF circulation (Lapras catheter). One prong remains in the third ventricle and one in the fourth, so that the catheter remains fixed. Seventy-seven cases were operated on. There were three deaths, one from meningitis, one from pulmonary atelectasis, and one from diffuse hemorrhage of the brainstem directly related to the surgical technique. As for morbidity, 1 patient neurologically deteriorated and became incapacitated; 5 cases presented Parinaud's syndrome, all without full postoperative recovery; 12 presented pseudomeningocele; and there was catheter migration in 4 cases, all of which had used catheters without prongs. As a final result, of the 77 patients, hydrocephalus was controlled in 39 of them, 30 required an external shunt, 3 died, and the result was not determined in 5 cases [26].

1.2.2 Third Ventriculostomy Through Craniotomy

Dandy, in 1922, described for the first time a third ventriculostomy technique through subfrontal access. It involved technically challenging surgery requiring the section of a healthy optic nerve. The interpeduncular cistern was reached laterally, and the posterior portion of the third ventricle floor was perforated. Six children were operated on by this technique [15]. In 1945, Dandy described a new subtemporal third ventriculostomy technique. The case involved 92 children undergoing this surgery, with a 12% mortality rate and control of hydrocephalus in 50% of the survivors, during a 7-year observation period [27]. In 1936, Stookey and Scarff described a new subfrontal third ventriculostomy technique called "puncture of the lamina terminalis and floor of the third ventricle." The most important and essential aspect of this technique is that both perforations are made in the midline, thus avoiding lesions of lateral structures such as the cavernous sinus, cranial nerves, and vessels in the region. In 1936, these authors published about 6 patients and, in 1951, about 34 patients, with a 15% mortality rate and control of hydrocephalus in 56% of the cases [28]. Another important case study of this technique reported a 2% mortality rate and 90% control of hydrocephalus in 230 operated patients during 7 years of follow-up [29]. Scarff carried out a review of the papers published by 19 authors reporting the results of 529 patients who underwent subfrontal and subtemporal third ventriculostomy. The review found 15% mortality and 70% control of hydrocephalus in an average period of 5 years of follow-up [14]. In 1968, Patterson and Bergland published their experience with 33 cases of third ventriculostomy using the subfrontal route, similar to that of Stookey and Scarff, but placing a perforated tube communicating the third ventricle and interpeduncular cistern. Of the 14 adults, 8 had relief for a period ranging from 31 months to 26 years. However, only 2 of the 13 children experienced relief [30]. Brocklehurst in 1974 described a technique in which he placed a catheter through the transcallosal route into the third ventricle and the interpeduncular cistern through the lamina terminalis and the floor. The catheter was attached to the cerebral falx, thus draining the cerebrospinal fluid from the third ventricle into the interhemispheric cisterns. Of the ten patients who underwent this technique, hydrocephalus was controlled in six, and of the remaining four, three died, and one required a ventriculoperitoneal shunt [31].

1.2.3   Stereotactic Third Ventriculostomy

In the 1970s, Poblete and Zamboni stated that the great number of techniques and devices used for treating hydrocephalus at the time showed that there was no definitive solution to the problem. They further stated that the treatment of choice for communicating hydrocephalus would be the ventriculoatrial shunt. In addition, from a theoretical point of view, third ventriculostomy to the interpeduncular cistern would be a rational method of treatment for obstructive hydrocephalus [32]. However, lack of precision inherent in the free-hand method has led them to consider the stereotactic technique more appropriate. The technique involves applying the stereotactic head frame and through a frontal trephine opening performing a ventriculography with positive contrast. The target determined by the lateral ventriculogram is located on the floor of the third ventricle, in the midline and posterior to the chiasmatic recess. A special cannula is introduced through the same craniotomy, with its correct positioning controlled by fluoroscopy. Once the floor has been perforated, air is injected into the cistern that allows checking the precision of the opening created. Ten patients were operated on with this technique. In all cases adequate drainage of the CSF was achieved. Three patients died due to the underlying causes of the obstruction (two of posterior fossa neoplasm and one of bacterial endocarditis resulting from valve infection). The autopsies showed the patency of the opening, in addition to the clinical progression of the survivors that allowed to observe its functioning [32]. Hoffman, in 1980, described a third ventriculostomy technique via the transcoronal approach using ventriculography as the basis of stereotactic orientation. He presented the results of 22 cases with a single complication, a transient palsy of the III nerve [33]. Kelly et al., in 1986, published about a technique for third ventriculostomy by the stereotactic method based on contrast-enhanced computed tomography. The patient is examined with the stereotactic head frame. A complicated localization system creates reference marks in each tomographic slice that allows calculating the position and slope of other slices in the stereotactic space. The surgeon chooses from the slices that pass through the interpeduncular cistern and the foramen of Monro points that exactly mark these structures. The computer calculates the position of these points in relation to the XYZ axes through special programs. This indicates the exact point of trepanation as well as the direction and depth of the puncture passing obviously through the foramen of Monro and interpeduncular cistern. The author further introduces an endoscope through the trepanation and confirms the direction of the needle using radiographs. These instruments are removed, and a leukotome is introduced to perform the perforation of the floor of the third ventricle at the place determined. Seven patients underwent this procedure, all with acquired hydrocephalus. All patients experienced relief of symptoms, and postoperative ventriculography with radioisotopes demonstrated communication of the third ventricle with the subarachnoid space in all cases. No complications and deaths were reported [34].

1.2.4 Percutaneous Third Ventriculostomy

In 1947, McNickle described a third ventriculostomy technique, using a coronal transfrontal approach and through the foramen of Monro to reach the interpeduncular cistern. The author initially injected dye into the lumbar subarachnoid space. He performed a trepanation on the right, at one-half to 1 inch from the midline, and at one-half to 1 inch posterior to the coronal suture. He inserted a needle (19G) through this trepanation in a direction slightly ahead of the temporomandibular joint and slightly medially (corner of the eye of the same side). Under radiological control, using anteroposterior and lateral radiographs, the needle was directed to the region immediately posterior to the posterior clinoid process, in the midline. The needle was moved side-by-side perforating the floor of the third ventricle, and if correctly applied, colored CSF previously injected into the lumbar space was collected. The author reported that in the first four cases, he introduced an endoscope into the lateral ventricle through a separate incision to guide the passage of the needle through the foramen of Monro. Using this method, he treated four cases of obstructive hydrocephalus, all achieving disease control, and three cases of communicating hydrocephalus, one of which remained unresolved [35]. Forjaz et al., in 1968, published a technique called "hypothalamic ventriculostomy with catheter." A trepanation was performed on the right, under local anesthesia, on the coronal suture, two fingers away from the midline. The lateral ventricle was punctured with a blunt needle, the foramen of Monro crossed, and the needle advanced to the floor of the third ventricle. The position of the needle was verified by cranial radiographs on axial and lateral views at a position 1–3 millimeters behind and above the tip projection of the posterior clinoid process. The needle was then advanced to the interpeduncular cistern and verified using lateral cranial radiography. Once properly positioned, the external part of the needle was removed, and a Nelaton 7F catheter, with several perforations in the distal portion, was introduced into the interpeduncular cistern guided by a metal stylet. After this metal stylet was removed, the catheter is closed at its distal end and fixed to the pericranium. This way, a communication between the third ventricle and the interpeduncular cistern, is established by the catheter in situ. The authors described 15 patients who underwent the procedure, 7 of them with neurocysticercosis, 5 with midline tumors, and 3 with hydrocephalus due to undetermined causes. All had obstructive hydrocephalus confirmed by pneumoventriculography. The technique provided relief in 12 cases, and 3 patients died [36]. Sayers and Kosnik, in 1976, imagined that third ventriculostomy could be applied to chronic patients dependent on external shunts, with many revisions. These patients theoretically could have subarachnoid spaces enlarged by functioning low-pressure valves prior to the procedure. They devised a procedure in which two leukotomes were introduced, one with a coronal approach and the other anterior. This way, the lamina terminalis and the floor of the third ventricle were opened. The procedure was performed under general anesthesia, with the third ventricle points marked by ventriculography, molds, and punctures guided by fluoroscopy and image amplifier. He used this technique in 46 pediatric patients, and 22 of these children exceeded the longest revision period for their valves. One child died of postoperative hemorrhage and hypothalamic injury, one had a permanent hypothalamic lesion, and three others had transient lesions [37]. Jacksche and Loew, in 1986, published the results of 79 patients undergoing third ventriculostomy by percutaneous coronal technique and guided by image amplifier in two planes. The catheter was advanced through the foramen of Monro, and the floor of the third ventricle perforated shortly after the posterior clinoid process. After reaching the cistern, 1 ml of contrast was injected to confirm the position. In patients with non-tumoral aqueductal stenosis and in patients with tumors with obstruction of the aqueduct, good results were achieved in 80% of the cases. Patients with a history of inflammatory diseases, those previously underwent shunt procedures, and patients with Dandy-Walker malformation did not respond well to the procedure. They also affirmed that after using cisternography to identify patients who had patent cisterns (among those with aqueductal stenosis), the failure rate decreased from 35% to 10% [38].

1.3   Development of Endoscopic Third Ventriculostomy

1.3.1   Pioneers of Neuroendoscopy

The era of neuroendoscopy began in 1910, when the American urologist Victor Darwin Lespinasse (1878–1946) made the first attempt to treat hydrocephalus by destroying the choroid plexus in two children using a cystoscope [39]. Later in 1922, Walter Edward Dandy (1886–1946) also used a cystoscope to visualize the ventricles and was able to inspect the lateral ventricle, the foramen of Monro, the choroid plexus, and even the blood vessels on the ventricular wall, thus coining the term "ventriculoscopy." Dandy also described an attempt to alleviate hydrocephalus using a small cystoscope, through a subfrontal approach by opening the lamina terminalis of the third ventricle. However, this technique was morbid, since one of the optic nerves was sacrificed for the approach. Dandy conducted this procedure a few times and stated that pneumoventriculography provided the same level of visualization and that endoscopy was not ready to replace traditional surgical methods in the treatment of hydrocephalus [15, 17, 40–42]. Dandy was the most important pioneer of neuroendoscopy, even devising the first ventriculoscope. At the same time, in the 1920s, the first endoscopic third ventriculostomy was performed by Mixter in 1923 [2].

1.3.2   Mixter: Summary Biography and the First ETV

Dr. William Jason Mixter (1880–1958) (Fig. 1.9) grew up in Boston, on his family farm in Berkshires. He attended the Massachusetts Institute of Technology, obtaining a degree in Biology, and started Harvard Medical School in 1902. After

Fig. 1.9 William Jason
Mixter (1880–1958).
(Reprinted from Decq et al.
[39]. With permission from
Elsevier)

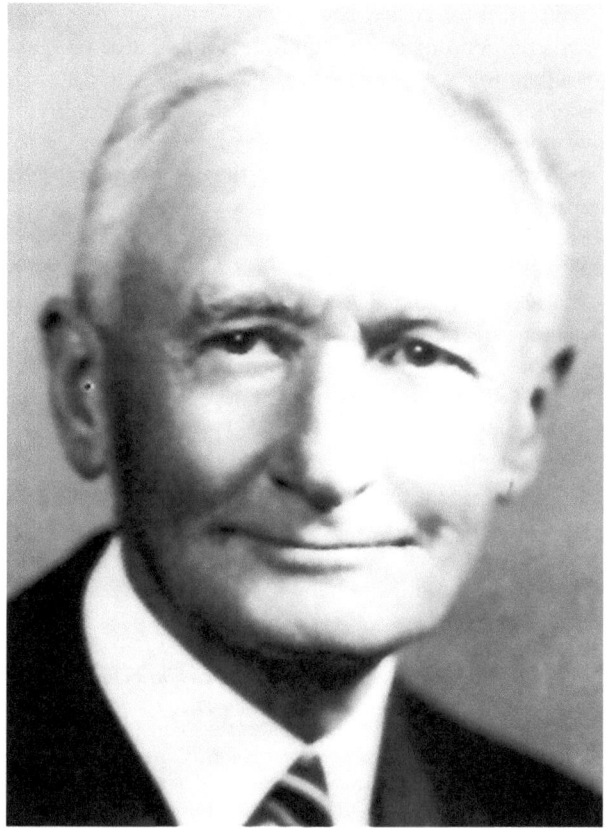

graduation, he began private medical practice in an office, joining his father and
brother. In 1915, Dr. Mixter went to France to serve in World War I as a civilian
surgeon 2 years before the United States entered the conflict. After a brief trip back
to Boston, he returned to France, this time in uniform as a military surgeon. A year
later, he was transferred to England and served as commander of Base Hospital
204 in Hursley Park during the great flu pandemic that broke out at the end of the
war. During this time, he demonstrated his skills as an administrator, dealing with
the difficult economic and administrative problems in times of war. Although he
practiced general surgery until 1920, Dr. Mixter's interest in neurosurgery dates
back to 1911, when he and his father designated two beds in Massachusetts General
Hospital especially for procedures developed by Horsley and Cushing. In 1933, he
was appointed Chief of Neurosurgery and in the following years convinced the hospital's trustees of the need for additional beds, better facilities in the operating room,
and a specific neurosurgery resident. In 1939, a separate neurosurgery department
was established with him as chief. Dr. Mixter retired in 1940, but resumed leading
the Neurosurgery Department from 1941 to 1946 during World War II, while his
successor, Dr. James C. White, was on active duty in the Navy. At that time,
Dr. Mixter also held the position of Senior Neurosurgery Consultant for the Surgeon

General of the Army. His great scientific interest was treatment of pain in the sympathetic nervous system and the spinal cord. His best-known work, performed in conjunction with Dr. Joseph Barr from the Orthopedics Department, involved the problem of low back pain with sciatic radiation. A prolific author, Dr. Mixter has written articles on a wide range of medical topics. In 1934, he and Dr. Barr coauthored the first paper defining the intervertebral disc protrusion syndrome. This article is still considered a classic. In addition, along with Walter Dandy and Max Peet, he coauthored neurosurgery sections for *Practice of Surgery* by Dean Lewis, as well as *Handbook of Health for Overseas Service* along with George Cheever Shattuck. Dr. Mixter was elected to the American Surgical Association in 1920 and was one of the original members of the Society of Neurological Surgeons. He was associated with many other medical societies and was also a member of the Massachusetts Institute of Technology Corporation and served as a trustee at the Massachusetts General Hospital. Throughout 20 years of neurosurgical practice, Dr. Mixter trained 28 young doctors in the art and science of neurosurgery. Many have developed their own training programs, thus disseminating the experience they gained with Dr. Mixer in the early days of neurosurgery at MGH [43]. Specifically in neuroendoscopy, Mixter performed the first endoscopic third ventriculostomy in 1923 in a 9-month-old baby [44].

> *"On February 6, 1923, under ether anaesthesia, an opening was made through the fontanelle in the right temporal region and the brain exposed. A small incision was made in the dura and a direct vision urethroscope passed into the ventricle. Under visual guidance, the urethroscope was passed through the dilated foramen of Monro and the third ventricle explored. The dilated aqueduct could be easily seen, but could not be entered with the urethroscope. Under visual guidance, a flexible sound was pushed through the floor of the third ventricle and the opening was enlarged by moving the sound from side to side until it was about 4 mm across. The edges of this opening immediately began to vibrate, apparently due to the passage of a current through the opening and this continued during the short period that the opening was under observation. The urethroscope was withdrawn and the dura and scalp closed with fine silk."*

1.3.3   Later Years

In 1923, Temple Fay (1895–1963) and Francis Grant (1891–1967) developed a method for capturing black and white images of the ventricles using a cystoscope (Fig. 1.10). The case report of a 10-month-old Italian boy illustrated an attempt to fenestrate the corpus callosum to treat hydrocephalus, but they failed to split the corpus callosum because of a malfunction in the cystoscope they were using. Although the procedure did not go as planned, they concluded that it was safe to view the ventricle using an endoscope without causing ventricular hemorrhage or other complications [45, 46]. Over 10 years later, in 1934, Tracy Putnam (1894–1975) introduced the "ventriculoscope" in order to perform the choroid plexectomy that

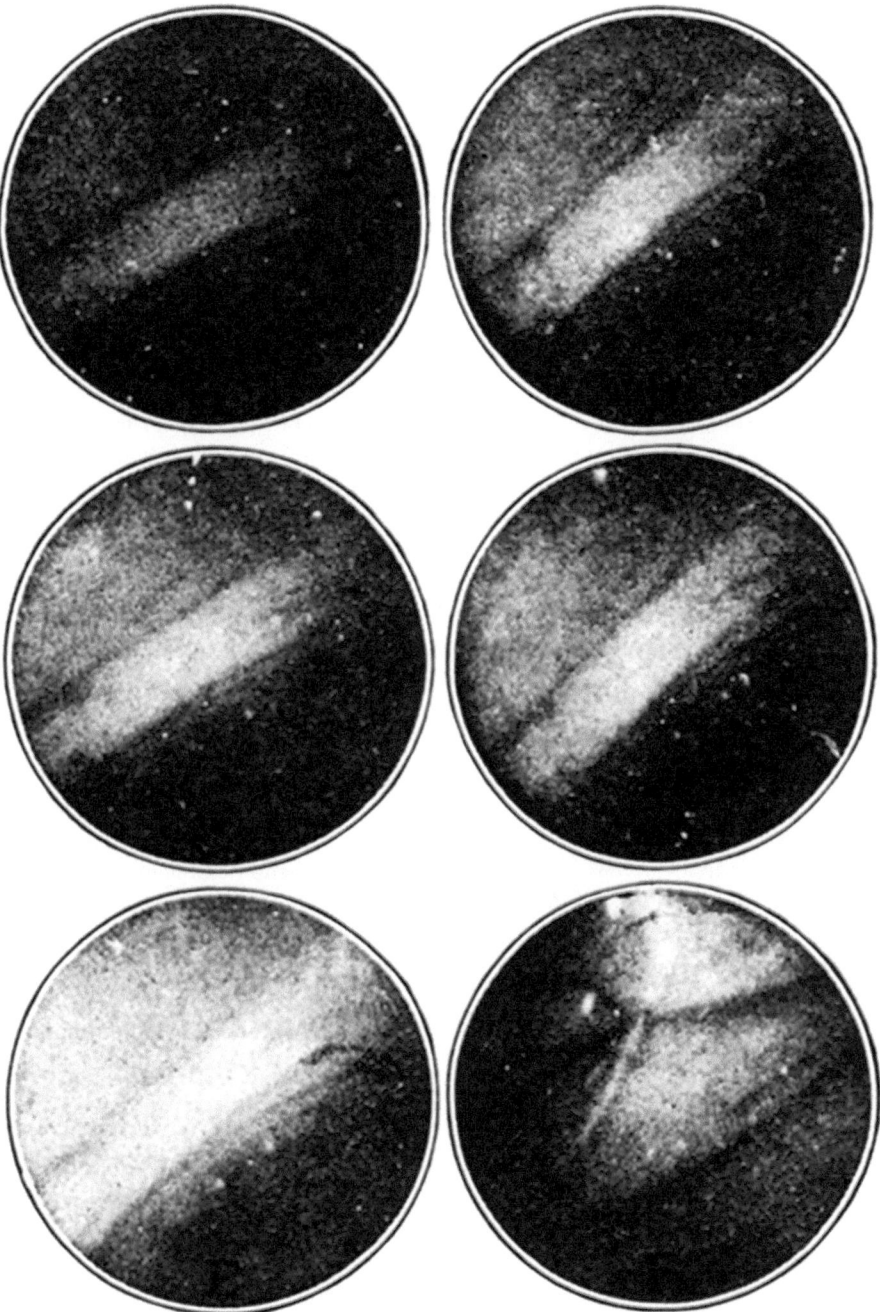

Fig. 1.10 First endoscopic images of the ventricles of 1923. (Reprinted from Fay and Grant [45])

Dandy had performed with the cystoscope. Putnam gave very specific details of his device and how it worked. He explained that it consisted of an optical glass rod with three grooves, one longitudinal groove for the light source and two other grooves for the diathermy electrodes. He went on to describe that his ventriculoscope came in two sizes; one was 10 cm long and 6 mm in diameter, while the other was 18 cm long and 7 mm in diameter. His initial experience was published in 1934 [46, 47]. In 1935, John Scarff (1898–1979) adapted an improved version of Putnam's ventriculoscope. While both shared the same concept, the devices were slightly different. Scarff's ventriculoscope had an irrigation system to maintain intraventricular pressure, thus preventing ventricular collapse. His device was also equipped with a flexible unipolar probe and a wide-angle lens for better viewing. Scarff also suggested that the opening into the third ventricle should be slightly more than just a puncture [46]. A new wave of development came from Europe in the 1960s. In 1961, Dereymaeker, van den Bergh, and Stroobandt adapted a new method for ventriculostomy, and fenestration of the lamina terminalis was performed using the light source itself. Their sample consisted of 15 patients, but only two of them had decreased ventricular size [39]. In the 1960s, the French neurosurgeon Gerard Guiot (1912–1998) revived the whole idea of neuroendoscopy after it was ostracized. His first endoscopic third ventriculostomy was successfully performed on August 8, 1962, in a 40-year-old man with a history of head trauma. The endoscope allowed Guiot to clearly see a tumor that was connected to the foramen of Monro, as well as a clear view of the lateral ventricle. Using a soft spatula, he was able to push the tumor into the third ventricle and perforate its floor. His second attempt was performed 1 year later on a child with hydrocephalus, using the same technique, and the patient's hydrocephalus was resolved after ventriculostomy. He continued to use this technique on several other occasions [39]. The next generation of neuroendoscopy would arrive in the 1970s based on an important contribution of the British physicist Harold Hopkins (1918–1994), whose innovative work paved the way for rigid and flexible endoscopes used today [46]. Takanori Fukushima (born in 1942) invented the "ventriculofiberscope," in 1973, and became the first neurosurgeon to use a flexible endoscope for ventriculostomy [48]. Around the same time, in England, Hugh Griffith (1930–1993) recommended the endoscopic procedure as a "first-line treatment for childhood hydrocephalus." He used Hopkins's rigid endoscope to perform third ventriculostomy, as well as choroid plexus coagulation to treat hydrocephalus [49]. In 1977, Michael Apuzzo (born in 1940) became the first to use a side-viewing wide-angled lens in neuroendoscopy [39]. Another development came in 1996, when Rieger et al. introduced the idea of using ultrasound to pass the endoscope into the third ventricle through the foramen of Monro. He described this technique as "accurate as the stereotactic technique, but faster and easier" [50]. In 1998, Veit Rohde et al. improved the use of stereotaxy in endoscopic third ventriculostomy, resulting in decreased postoperative morbidity [51]. Entering the new millennium, there was another addition of technology to the procedure. In 2002, neuroendoscopy was used in conjunction with neuronavigation to decrease vascular injury during the procedure, and in 2004, the first instance of a robot used in a third ventriculostomy was reported [52, 53]. One of the most recent contributions to the development of ETV came from

Benjamin Warf of Boston Children's Hospital. He reported on the combination of ETV and choroid plexus cauterization (CPC) in order to produce better results in the treatment of hydrocephalus, especially in developing countries, where shunt procedures can be dangerous due to a lack of resources to revise a shunt after malfunction or infection. Based on this assumption, Warf conducted his EVT/CPC trials in East Africa from June 2001 to December 2004. His initial results in 2005 suggested that ETV/CPC was better than ETV alone in patients under 1 year of age, especially those with myelomeningocele and "non-postinfectious" hydrocephalus. In 2012, after several trials, it became clear that children below 1 year of age with congenital aqueductal stenosis would benefit the most from ETV/CPC. In 2014, Warf validated his results from Uganda by conducting ETV/CPC trials in North American patients, and the results were consistent with his previous experience. He also found that ETV/CPC carried a lower postoperative infection or malfunction risk compared to shunt procedures, thus offering a substantial cost-effectiveness advantage [54–56].

References

1. Torack RM. Historical aspects of normal and abnormal brain fluids. I Cerebrospinal fluids. Arch Neurol. 1982a;39:197–201.
2. Dezena RA. Atlas of endoscopic neurosurgery of the third ventricle. Basic principles for ventricular approaches and essential intraoperative anatomy. Cham: Springer International Publishing AG; 2017. https://doi.org/10.1007/978-3-319-50068-3-1.
3. Siraisi NG. Medieval and early renaissance medicine: an introduction to knowledge and practice. Chicago: The University of Chicago Press; 1990.
4. Keele KD. Leonardo da Vinci's influence on Renaissance anatomy. Med Hist. 1964;8:360–70.
5. Torack RM. Historical aspects of normal and abnormal brain fluids. II Hydrocephalus. Arch Neurol. 1982b;39:276–9.
6. Milhorat TH. The third circulation revisited. J Neurosurg. 1975;42:628–45.
7. Schroeck L. De infante hydrocephalo. Maladies Neurologie in Miscellanea curiosa... Observationes Medico-Physico-Anatomico-Botanico-Mathematicas, t. 22 (1696), p. 238 Enfant hydrocéphale.
8. Ruysch F. Thesaurus anatomicus secundus. Collection: de anatomische preparaten van Frederik Ruysch. (1638–1731). Amsterdam, 1702 Tabula III - Thes. II.
9. Pacchioni A. Disquisitio anatomicae de dura e meningis... Leipzig Acta Eruditorum, 1703.
10. Morgagni GB. De sedibus, et causis morborum per anatomen indagatis libri quinque. Typographia Remondiniana, 1761.
11. Davis M, Loukas M, Tubbs RS. Jean Cruveilhier and his contributions to understanding childhood hydrocephalus, Chiari II malformation, and spina bifida. Childs Nerv Syst. 2018;34(9):1613–5. https://doi.org/10.1007/s00381-017-3529-4.
12. Cruveilhier J. Anatomie pathologique du corps humain. J. B. Baillière 1829–42, Paris;1829.
13. Dandy WE. Diagnosis and treatment of hydrocephalus resulting from strictures of the aqueduct of Sylvius. Surg Gynecol Obstet. 1920;31:340–58.
14. Scarff JE. Treatment of hydrocephalus by operations not requiring mechanical tubes or valves. In: Workshop in hydrocephalus. Philadelphia: Proceedings: The Children Hospital of Philadelphia; 1965. p. 38–78.
15. Dandy WE. An operative procedure for hydrocephalus. Bull Johns Hopk Hosp. 1922;33:189–90.

16. Nulsen FE, Spitz EB. Treatment of hydrocephalus by direct shunt from ventricle to jugular vein. Surg Forum. 1951;2:399–403.
17. Demerdash A, Rocque BG, Johnston J, Rozzelle CJ, Yalcin B, Oskouian R, et al. Endoscopic third ventriculostomy: a historical review. Br J Neurosurg. 2017;31(1):28–32. https://doi.org/1 0.1080/02688697.2016.1245848.
18. Rekate HL. Does it matter which shunt is used? Crit Rev Neurosurg. 1996;6:57–63.
19. Milhorat TH, Hammock MK, Di Chiro G. The subarachnoid space in congenital obstructive hydrocephalus. Part 1: Cisternographic findings. J Neurosurg. 1971;35:1–6.
20. Naidich TP, Mclone DG. Radiographic classification and gross morphologic features of hydrocephalus. In: Hoffman H, Epstein F, editors. Disorders of the developing nervous system: diagnosis and treatment. London: Blackwell Scientific Publications; 1986. p. 505–39.
21. Leksell L. A surgical procedure for atresia of the aqueduct of Sylvius. Acta Psychiatr Neurol. 1949;24:559–68.
22. Elvidge AR. Treatment of obstructive lesions of the aqueduct of Sylvius and fourth ventricle by interventriculostomy. J Neurosurg. 1966;24:11–26.
23. Cuatico W, Richardson NK. Transcutaneous therapeutic canalization of aqueductal stenosis in a hydrocephalic; case report and technical note. Acta Neurochir. 1979;47:181–6.
24. Avman N, Dinçer C. Venous malformation of the aqueduct of Sylvius treated by interventriculostomy: 15 years follow-up. Acta Neurochir. 1980;52:219–24.
25. Backlund EO, Grepe A, Lunsford D. Stereotaxic reconstruction of the aqueduct of Sylvius. J Neurosurg. 1981;55:800–10.
26. Lapras CL, Bret JD, Patet JD, Huppert J, Honorato D. Hydrocephalus and aqueduct stenosis. Direct surgical treatment by interventriculostomy (aqueduct cannulation). J Neurosurg Sci. 1986;30:47–53.
27. Dandy WE. Diagnosis and treatment of strictures of the aqueduct of Sylvius (causing hydrocephalus). Arch Surg. 1945;51(1):14.
28. Scarff JE. Treatment of obstructive hydrocephalus by puncture of the lamina terminalis and floor of the third ventricle. J Neurosurg. 1951;8:204–13.
29. Guillaume J, Mazars G. Indications et résultats de la ventriculostomie sus-optique dans l'hydrocéphalie de l'adulte. Rev Neurol. 1950;82:421–4.
30. Patterson RH, Bergland RM. The selection of patients for third ventriculostomy based on experience with 33 operations. J Neurosurg. 1968;29:252–4.
31. Brocklehurst G. Trans-calosal third ventriculo-chiasmatic cisternostomy: a new approach to hydrocephalus. Surg Neurol. 1974;2:109–14.
32. Poblette M, Zamboni R. Stereotaxic third ventriculocisternostomy. Confinia Neurol. 1979;37:150–5.
33. Hoffman HJ, Harwood-Nash D, Gilday DL. Percutaneous third ventriculostomy in the management of noncommunicating hydrocephalus. Neurosurgery. 1980;7:313–21.
34. Kelly JP, Goers S, Kall BA, Kispert DB. Computed tomography-based stereotactic third ventriculostomy: technical note. Neurosurgery. 1986;18:791–9.
35. Mcnickle HF. The surgical treatment of hydrocephalus: a simple method of performing third ventriculostomy. Brit J Surg. 1947;34:302–7.
36. Forjaz S, Martelli N, Latuf N. Hypothalamic ventriculostomy with catheter: technical note. J Neurosurg. 1968;29:655–9.
37. Sayers MP, Kosnik EJ. Percutaneous third ventriculostomy: experience and technique. Childs Brain. 1976;2:24–30.
38. Jaksche H, Loew F. Burr hole third ventriculo-cisternostomy: an unpopular but effective procedure for treatment of certain forms of occlusive hydrocephalus. Acta Neurochir. 1986;79:48–51.
39. Decq P, Schroeder HW, Fritsch M, Cappabianca P. A history of ventricular neuroendoscopy. World Neurosurg. 2013;79(2Suppl):S14.e1–6. https://doi.org/10.1016/j.wneu.2012.02.034.
40. Dandy WE. Cerebral ventriculoscopy. Bull Johns Hopkins Hosp. 1922;33:189.

41. Scarff JE. Third ventriculostomy as the rational treatment of obstructive hydrocephalus. J Pediatr. 1935;6:870–1.
42. Kretzer RM, Crosby RW, Rini DA, Tamargo RJ. Dorcas Hager Padget: neuroembryologist and neurosurgical illustrator trained at Johns Hopkins. J Neurosurg. 2004;100(4):719–30. https://doi.org/10.3171/jns.2004.100.4.0719.
43. MGH Neurosurgery Alumni Society. William Jason Mixter. 2010; Available at: https://alumni.neurosurgery.mgh.harvard.edu/mixter.htm.
44. Mixter WJ. Ventriculoscopy and puncture of the floor of the third ventricle. Boston Med & Surg J. 1923;188:277–8.
45. Fay T, Grant FC. Ventriculoscopy and intraventricular photography in internal hydrocephalus: report of case. J Am Med Assoc. 1923;80(7):461–3.
46. Geiger M, Cohen AT. The history of neuroendoscopy. In: Cohen A, Haines SJ, editors. Concepts in Neurosurgery Vol 7: minimally invasive techniques in neurosurgery. Baltimore: Williams & Wilkins; 1995. p. 1–13.
47. Putnam TJ. Treatment of hydrocephalus by endoscopic coagulation of the choroid plexus: description of a new instrument and preliminary report of results. New Engl J Med. 1934;210(26):1373–6.
48. Fukushima T, Ishijima B, Hirakawa K, Nakamura N, Sano K. Ventriculofiberscope: a new technique for endoscopic diagnosis and operation: technical note. J Neurosurg. 1973;38(2):251–6.
49. Griffith HB, Jamjoom AB. The treatment of childhood hydrocephalus by choroid plexus coagulation and artificial cerebrospinal fluid perfusion. Brit J Neurosurg. 1990;4(2):95–100.
50. Rieger A, Rainov NG, Sanchin L, Schöpp G, Burkert W. Ultrasound-guided endoscopic fenestration of the third ventricular floor for non-communicating hydrocephalus. Min Inv Neurosurg. 1996;39(1):17–20.
51. Rohde V, Reinges MHT, Krombach GA, Gilsbach JM. The combined use of image-guided frameless stereotaxy and neuroendoscopy for the surgical management of occlusive hydrocephalus and intracranial cysts. Brit J Neurosurg. 1998;12(6):531–8.
52. Schmitt PJ, Jane JA Jr. A lesson in history: the evolution of endoscopic third ventriculostomy. Neurosurg Focus. 2012;33(2):E11.
53. Sgouros S. Neuroendoscopy: current status and future trends. Berlin: Springer; 2013.
54. Stone SS, Warf BC. Combined endoscopic third ventriculostomy and choroid plexus cauterization as primary treatment for infant hydrocephalus: a prospective North American series: Clinical article. J Neurosurg: Pediatrics. 2014;14(5):439–46.
55. Warf BC. Comparison of endoscopic third ventriculostomy alone and combined with choroid plexus cauterization in infants younger than 1 year of age: a prospective study in 550 African children. J Neurosurg. 2005;103(6 Suppl):475–81.
56. Warf BC, Tracy S, Mugamba J. Long-term outcome for endoscopic third ventriculostomy alone or in combination with choroid plexus cauterization for congenital aqueductal stenosis in African infants: Clinical article. J Neurosurg Pediatrics. 2012;10(2):108–11.

Chapter 2
Anatomy and Physiology of the Ventricular System

2.1 Anatomy

2.1.1 Historical Milestones of the Ventricular Anatomy

It is believed that the human ventricular system was first described in the third century BC by the Greeks Erasistratus (ca. 304 BC ca. 250 BC) and Herophilus (ca. 335 BC ca. 280 BC), who were allowed to perform dissections and vivisections in humans [1]. Claudius Galen (ca. 129 ca. 217) established that the ventricles were responsible for storing the animal spirit (*pneumapsychikon*), which would be the active element of the brain and nerves. At the time, Galen, who was gladiators' physician, observed that when a traumatic injury affected the ventricles, death would never occur, even if sensitivity and strength were affected. Furthermore, imagination, reason, and memory, considered the three constituents of the human intellect, could be affected separately by such lesions [2, 3]. From these ancient citations, together with initial notions of Christian authorities, the Cell Doctrine was established, which tried to elucidate some aspects of cerebral physiology from the ventricles. In the fourth century, the Byzantine physician Poseidon overhauled Galen's theories, probably becoming the first to report on notions regarding brain location, stating that anterior brain lesions afflict imagination, medial brain lesions afflict reason, and posterior regions afflict memory [3, 4]. At the same time, other church officials, particularly Nemesius, bishop of Emesa (ca. 390) and St. Augustine (354–430), sought to conceptualize the nonmaterial nature of the soul, located within the ventricles. The Cell Doctrine remained in force throughout the Middle Ages. What is now known as lateral ventricles were considered a single cavity, the first cell in its anterior part received external and other impulses from the rest of the body, characterizing common sense (sensus communis). From this region, imagination (*imaginativa*) and abstractions (*fantasia*) were created in the posterior part of the first cell. The second cell (currently the third ventricle) was the locus of cognitive processes, such as reason (*ratio*), judgment (*aestimativa*), and thought (*cogitativa*). The function of the

© Springer Nature Switzerland AG 2020
R. A. Dezena, *Endoscopic Third Ventriculostomy*,
https://doi.org/10.1007/978-3-030-28657-6_2

posterior cell (currently the fourth ventricle) would be the memory center (*memorativa*) [3, 5, 6]. Such concepts remained dogmatic until the Renaissance, when they began to be seriously questioned, with the emergence of more precise anatomical descriptions. Curiously, throughout the Dark Ages, there were only unillustrated descriptions of the Cell Doctrine. It was during the Renaissance that the first illustrations began to appear (Fig. 2.1). The great master of the Renaissance, Leonardo da Vinci (1452–1519), was the first to combine his experiences as an artist and a deep connoisseur of anatomy. He represents a true transition and the essence of the Renaissance spirit, as he created illustrations of the Cell Doctrine and, in contrast, more accurate illustrations of the ventricular cavity from his own dissections [8–11] (Figs. 2.2 and 2.3). In 1543, the watershed of the history of anatomy emerged, considered by many authors as a major book on the history of science: *De humani corporis fabrica libri septem* or *De humani corporis fabrica*, or simply *Fabrica*, written by the Belgian Andreas Vesalius (1514–1564), considered the "father of modern anatomy" [15]. This work contained incredible anatomical details of the ventricles (Fig. 2.4). In 1663, a Dutch anatomist named Franz de le Boë (1614–1672) or *Franciscus Sylvius* in Latinized form also described the cerebral aqueduct [16].

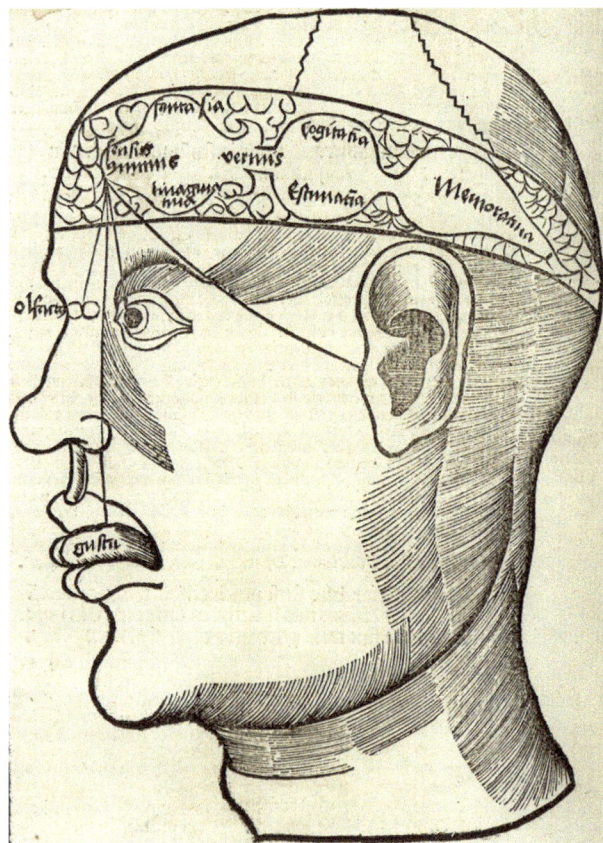

Fig. 2.1 Representation of the senses and the faculties inside, according to the Cell Doctrine [7]. (Reprinted from Reisch [7])

Fig. 2.2 "The Layers of the Scalp Compared with an Onion" (ca.1490–1492). Still relying on the Cell Doctrine theory, the master Leonardo da Vinci drew the brain in pen and ink according to the accepted notion of three cells, while the rest of the head was drawn realistically [12]. (Reprinted from Vinci et al. [12])

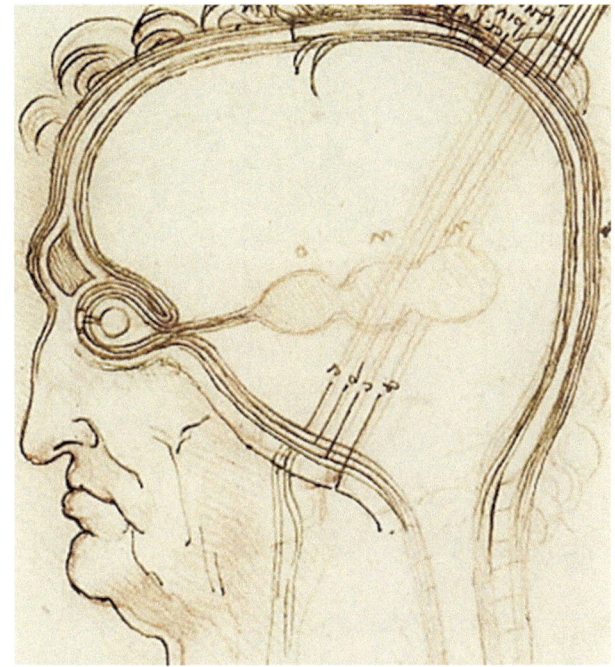

Fig. 2.3 "Study of brain physiology" (ca. 1508). Drawing in pen and ink by the master Leonardo da Vinci after his study of ox brain injections. This rendering of the human brain, ventricles, visual pathways, and skull base reveals Leonardo's dissection experience and his break from traditional scholasticism, at least as far as personal experience and depiction are concerned [13, 14]. (Image courtesy of History of Science Collections, University of Oklahoma Libraries)

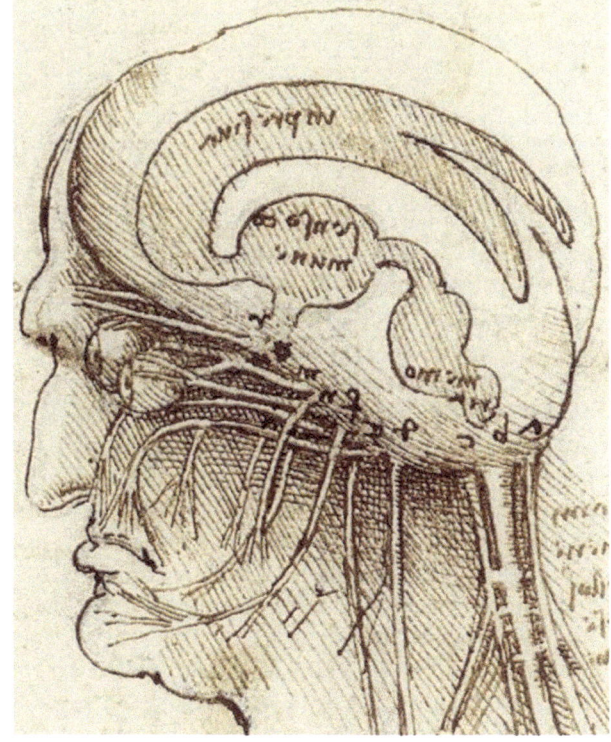

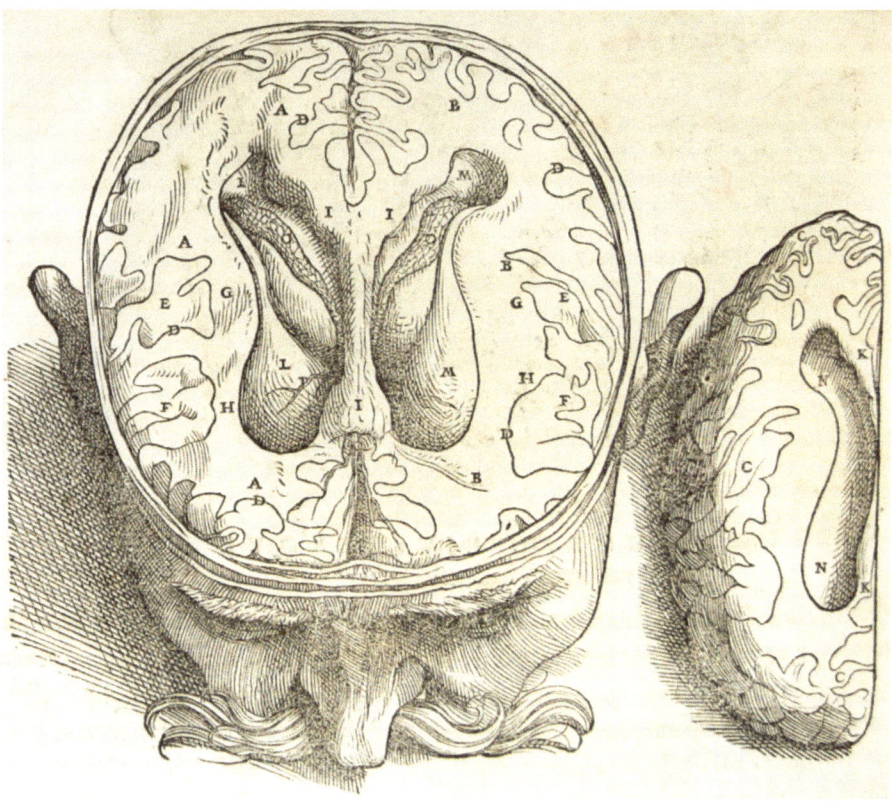

Fig. 2.4 The lateral ventricles from Fabrica, in its first edition of 1543 [15]. (Image courtesy of History of Science Collections, University of Oklahoma Libraries)

Curiously, even after the accurate descriptions of the Renaissance, doubts remained as to the true content of the ventricular cavity, whether it was liquid or gaseous. This doubt finally came to an end in 1764 by the Italian Domenico Felice Antonio Cotugno (1736–1822), who discovered the cerebrospinal fluid (CSF). The interventricular foramen was described in 1783 and is credited to Scottish Alexander Monro Secundus (1733–1817) [2]. The finding of continuity between ventricular cavity and subarachnoid space was confirmed by the French neurologist and experimental physiologist François Jean Magendie (1783–1855), at the medial region of the fourth ventricle, now known as the foramen of Magendie or median aperture of the fourth ventricle [17]. Other communication-related findings were made by the German anatomist Hubert von Luschka (1820–1875) in 1855, at the University of Tübingen. Such communications were known as lateral apertures of the fourth ventricle, or simply, foramina of Luschka [18]. Without a doubt, the main descriptions of the ventricles and CSF system are completed through the work of Axel Key (1832–1901) and Magnus Gustaf Retzius (1842–1919). In this work, which earned Retzius a professorship in histology at the Karolinska Institute, they injected colored gelatin into

Fig. 2.5 General aspect and topographic relationship of the ventricular system and the encephalon and head. (Reprinted from Dezena [42]. with permission from Springer Nature)

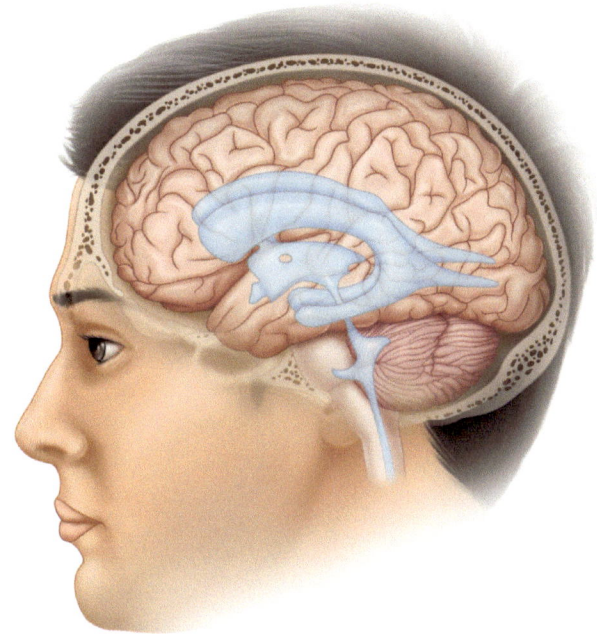

cadavers and showed that gelatin flows through arachnoid granulations, also called arachnoid villi or pacchionian granulations, into the superior sagittal sinus [19].

2.1.2   Basic Ventricular Anatomy

The ventricular system is divided into lateral, third, and fourth ventricles. The lateral ventricles connect to the third ventricle via the foramen of Monro, and the third ventricle connects to the fourth ventricle via the cerebral aqueduct (Figs. 2.5 and 2.6). Detailed knowledge of the anatomy of the lateral ventricles and the third ventricle is crucial for main ventricular endoscopic procedures. Each lateral ventricle has a frontal (anterior) horn, body, atrium, occipital (posterior) horn, and temporal (inferior) horn, and each of these parts has a roof, floor, and anterior, medial, and lateral walls [20, 21]. These boundaries can be found in Fig. 2.7. The third ventricle is a narrow midline cavity located at the center of the ventricular system. It communicates with the lateral ventricles through the foramen of Monro on its anterosuperior aspect and with the cerebral aqueduct on its posteroinferior aspect. The roof of the third ventricle forms a gentle upward arc, extending from the foramen of Monro anteriorly to the suprapineal recess posteriorly. It has four layers from superior to inferior: a neural layer formed by the fornix, superior membrane of the tela choroidea, vessels (lateral posterior choroidal arteries and internal cerebral veins), and inferior membrane of the tela choroidea [2]. The anterior half of the floor is

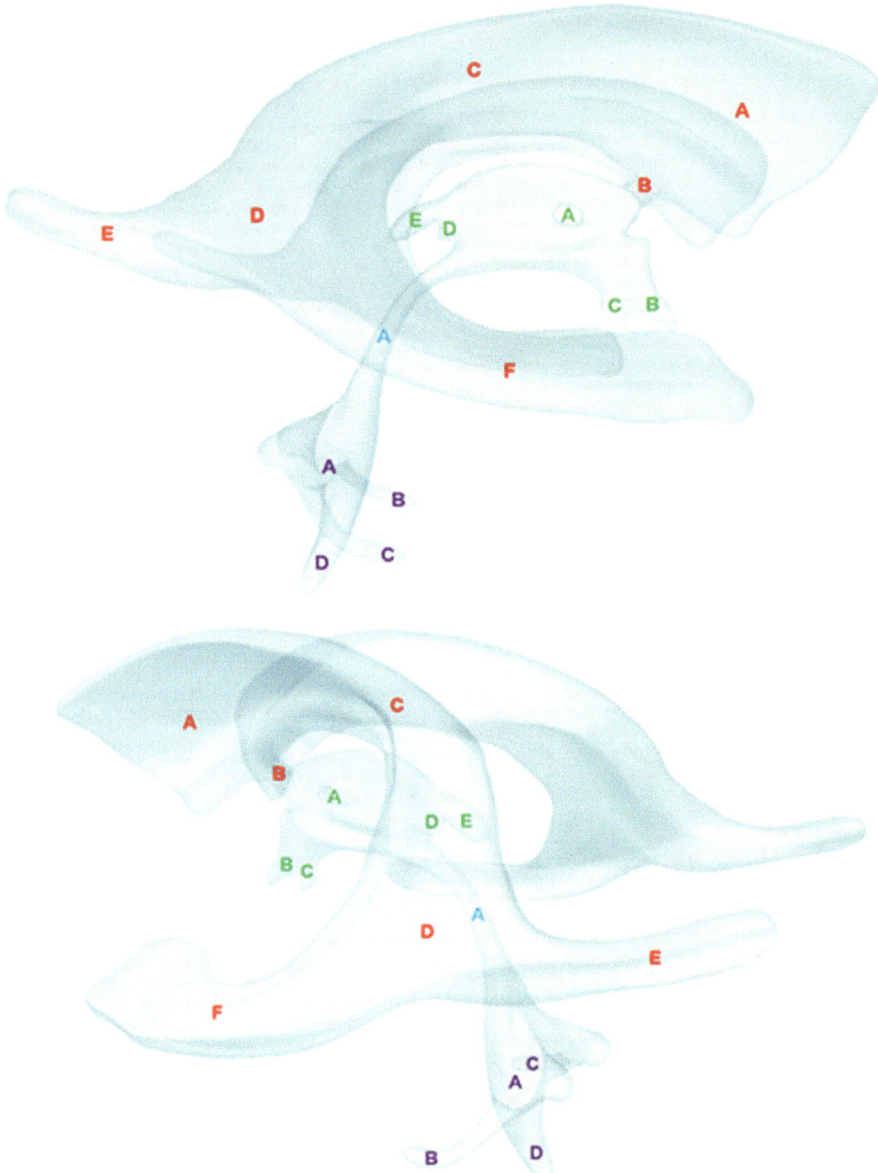

Fig. 2.6 The ventricular system in right lateral view (above) and left oblique lateral view (below). Lateral ventricle (in red): frontal horn (A), foramen of Monro (B), body (C), atrium (D), occipital horn (E), temporal horn (F). Third ventricle (in green): interthalamic adhesion (A), optic recess (B), infundibular recess (C), pineal recess (D), suprapineal recess (E). Cerebral aqueduct (in blue) (A). Fourth ventricle (in purple): fourth ventricle (A); left lateral recess and left lateral aperture of Luschka (B), right lateral recess and right lateral aperture of Luschka (C), median aperture of Magendie (D). (Reprinted from Dezena [42]. with permission from Springer Nature)

Lateral Ventricle	Roof	Floor	Anterior wall	Medial wall	Lateral wall
FRONTAL HORN	Genu of the corpus callosum	Rostrum of the corpus callosum	Genu of the corpus callosum	Septum pellucidum Columns of the fornix	Head of the caudate nucleus
BODY	Body of the corpus callosum	Thalamus		Septum pellucidum Body of the fornix	Body of the caudate nucleus Thalamus
ATRIUM	Body, splenium and tapetum of the corpus callosum	Collateral trigone	Crus of the fornix Pulvinar of the thalamus	Bulb of the corpus callosum Calcar avis	Tail of the caudate nucleus Tapetum of the corpus callosum
OCCIPITAL HORN	Tapetum of the corpus callosum	Collateral trigone		Bulb of the corpus callosum Calcar avis	Tapetum of the corpus callosum
TEMPORAL HORN	Thalamus Tail of the caudate nucleus Tapetum of the corpus callosum	Hippocampus Collateral eminence	Amygdala	Choroidal fissure	Tapetum of the corpus callosum

Fig. 2.7 Regions and limits of the lateral ventricle

Roof	Floor	Anterior wall	Posterior wall	Lateral wall
Body and crus of the fornix, hippocampal commissure	Optic chiasm	Columns of the fornix	Suprapineal recess	Thalamus
Tela choroidea and vessels (medial posterior choroidal artery and internal cerebral vein)	Infundibular recess	Foramen fo Monro	Habenular commissure	Hypothalamus
	Tuber cinereum	Anterior commissure	Pineal body and pineal recess	Columns of the fornix
	Mammillary bodies	Lamina terminalis	Posterior commissure	
	Posterior perforated substance	Optic recess	Cerebral aqueduct	
	Tegmentum of the mesencephalon	Optic chiasm		

Fig. 2.8 Regions and limits of the third ventricle

formed by diencephalic structures, and the posterior half is formed by mesencephalic structures [2, 21, 22]. The structures that constitute the floor include, from anterior to posterior, the optic chiasm, the infundibular recess, the tuber cinereum, the mammillary bodies, the posterior perforated substance, and the midbrain tegmentum located above the medial aspect of the cerebral peduncles. The lateral walls are formed by the thalamus, the hypothalamus, and the columns of the fornix. The posterior wall, from top to bottom, is formed by the suprapineal recess, the habenular commissure, the pineal body and its recess, the posterior commissure, and the cerebral aqueduct [21, 22]. The boundaries can be found in Fig. 2.8.

2.2   Physiology of Cerebrospinal Fluid (CSF) Circulation

It is assumed that most CSF circulating within the ventricles comes from the choroid plexus, but there is still controversy surrounding this issue [23]. Other CSF production sites, such as the cerebral parenchyma, are currently described as contributing to the total amount of circulating CSF [23, 24] (Fig. 2.9). The CSF formation rate in humans is 0.3–0.4 ml/min, with the total volume of CSF being approximately 90–150 ml in adults [25]. In addition, it had long been assumed that CSF was flowing from the lateral and third ventricles, areas with higher concentrations of choroid plexus, reaching the fourth ventricle via the cerebral aqueduct and finally the subarachnoid space through the foramina of Magendie and Luschka, being absorbed into venous blood at the arachnoid granulation level (Figs. 2.10, 2.11, and 2.12). This classic concept, known as the third circulation, which originated from animal studies, is also questioned today [23, 26]. In addition to its classical mechanical damping function, reducing apparent brain weight, it is now known that CSF is also rich in nutrients, including amino acids, vitamins, minerals, proteins, and ions in varying concentrations, depending on the stage of development [27, 28]. Today, there is great scientific evidence that CSF also plays an important role in the development and embryonic organization of the central nervous system through neuroendocrine communication [29, 30]. The ventricles are lined with ependymal cells, a single-layer tissue of ciliated cells called ependymocytes, which are in direct contact with cerebrospinal fluid [31]. Propulsion for circulation of cerebrospinal fluid results from macroscopic phenomena, such as pulsation of the choroid plexus and the beating of the ventricular wall, both due to cardiac systole. At the microscopic level, ciliary beating of the ependymocytes takes place [32] (Figs. 2.13 and 2.14). This ciliary movement occurs periodically, generating CSF flow in the vicinity of the ventricular wall [33]. It is proposed that this flow induced by ciliary beating eliminates small debris from the ventricular wall and has the effect of diluting substances, particularly in the third ventricle [34]. Genetic mutations affecting ciliary movement may be associated with

Fig. 2.9 Production sites and absorption routes of CSF. (Reprinted from Di Rocco [24]. With permission from Springer Nature)

Production sites
Choroid plexus
Extra-choroidal sites
  1. Ventricular ependyma
  2. Subarachnoid space
  3. Pia-arachnoid capillary
  4. Brain parenchyma
Absorption routes
Arachnoid villi→superior sagittal sinus
Extra-arachnoid villus sites
  1. Ventricular ependyma→subependymal vein
  2. Leptomeninges→cortical vein
  3. Pia-arachnoid capillary→venous system
  4. Choroid plexus→deep venous system
  5. Perineural space→lymphatic channel

Fig. 2.10 Traditional third circulation model of CSF pathway. CSF is produced by the choroid plexuses, from where it moves from the lateral ventricles into the third and fourth ventricles. It then flows across the surface of the brain and down the spinal canal (moving from the back to front of the canal). CSF is then reabsorbed by the arachnoid granulations back into the bloodstream. (Reprinted from Dezena [42]. with permission from Springer Nature)

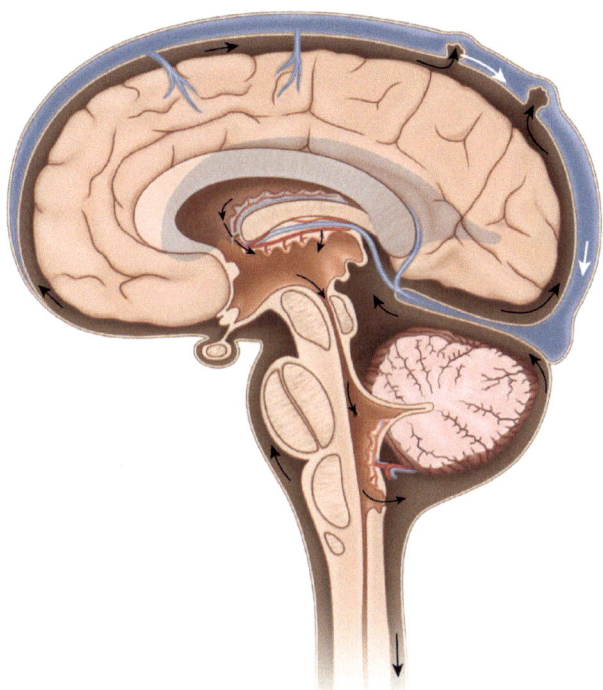

Fig. 2.11 Traditional third circulation model of CSF pathway ending in the arachnoid granulation, and later flowing toward the superior sagittal sinus. (Reprinted from Dezena [42]. with permission from Springer Nature)

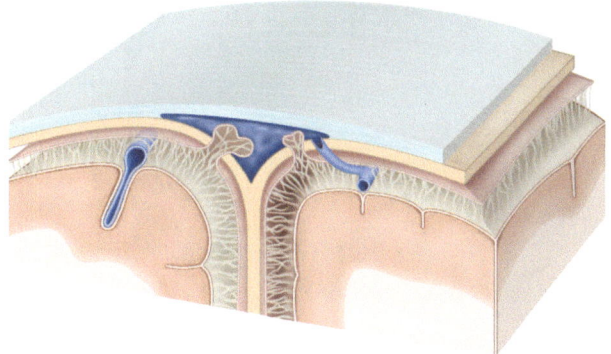

hydrocephalus [35–37]. Historically, it has always been argued that the absorption of CSF into the circulating blood is indeed more remarkable in the arachnoid granulation [38–40]. This notion is based on the first experiments performed by Key and Retzius, in which they injected colored gelatin into human cadavers. In fact, the distribution of the dye was observed throughout the CSF system, as well as its passage to the arachnoid granulation toward the venous sinuses [19]. However, their

Fig. 2.12 Arachnoid
granulation in detail. In fact,
arachnoid granulation is an
expansion, through the dura,
of the subarachnoid space to
the venous system.
(Reprinted from Dezena [42].
with permission from
Springer Nature)

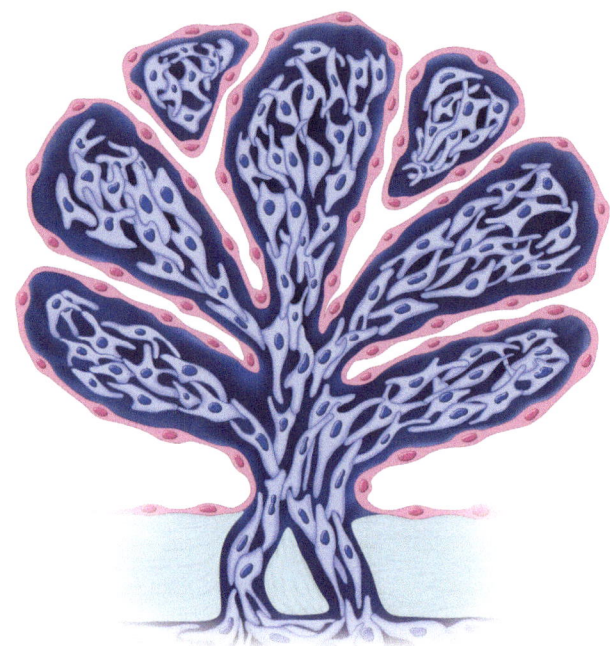

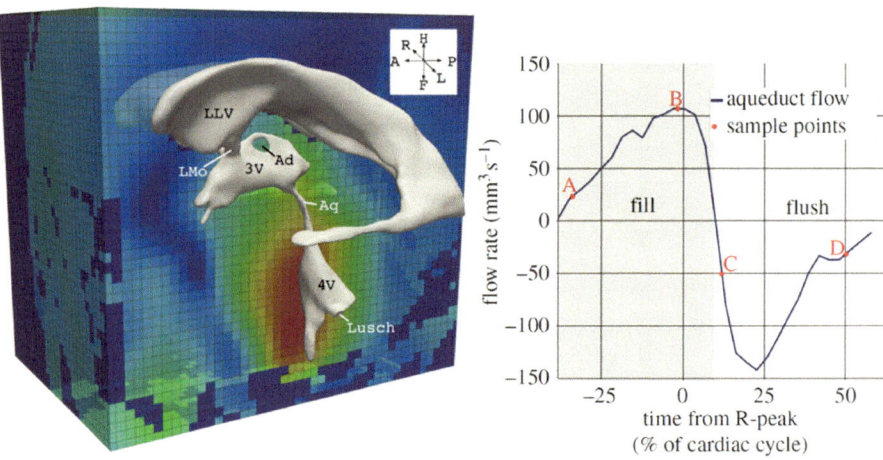

Fig. 2.13 In vivo data obtained with magnetic resonance imaging (MRI). On the right the ventricular geometry extracted from anatomical MR images is overlaid on the MRI displacement field. On the left, the CSF flow rate through the aqueduct is reconstructed from the two-dimensional phase contrast gradient echo sequence and the four sample points (A–D). Note that the electrocardiogram R-peak is used to define the start of the cardiac cycle. Points A and B are in the fill period where the flow through the aqueduct is oriented in the cranial direction, whereas points C and D correspond to the flush period where the CSF flow is in the caudal direction. Abbreviations: LLV left lateral ventricle, LMo left foramen of Monro, Ad interthalamic adhesion, 3V third ventricle, Aq cerebral aqueduct, 4V fourth ventricle, Lusch foramen of Luschka. (Reprinted from Siyahhan et al. [32]. With permission from Royal Society Publishing)

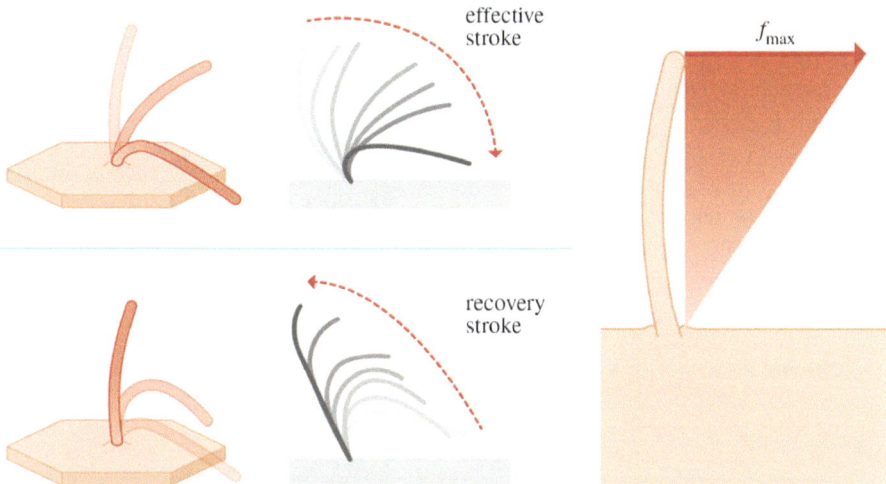

Fig. 2.14 Schematic of a beating ependymal cilium. The beating motion consists of an effective and a recovery stroke. The action of the cilia is accounted for via body forces acting on the CSF. The fmax (maximum force density) is determined empirically by matching the induced fluid velocity to experimental measurements. (Reprinted from Siyahhan et al.[32]. With permission from Royal Society Publishing)

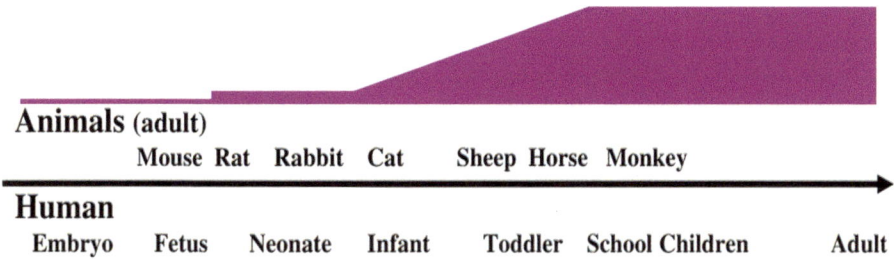

Fig. 2.15 Ontogenesis of arachnoid granulation in humans compared with other animals Oi S. (Reprinted from Di Rocco [24]. With permission from Springer Nature)

results were disputed because the gelatin was injected at a pressure of 60 mmHg, which could have caused a rupture in the arachnoid granulation [41]. Since then, other means of absorption of cerebrospinal fluid have been argued. The arachnoid granulation has a developmental mechanism in humans, comparable to other animals that are lower on the phylogenetic scale [24] (Fig. 2.15). During pregnancy, the fetus has virtually no arachnoid granulations, which can be compared to a mouse. They begin to develop from birth and are equivalent to a mouse and a rabbit. After 1 year of age, they develop greatly, gradually reaching a size similar to that of a cat, a sheep, and a horse and, finally at school age, similar to that of a monkey. During the immature period of the brain, the CSF absorption mechanism is not

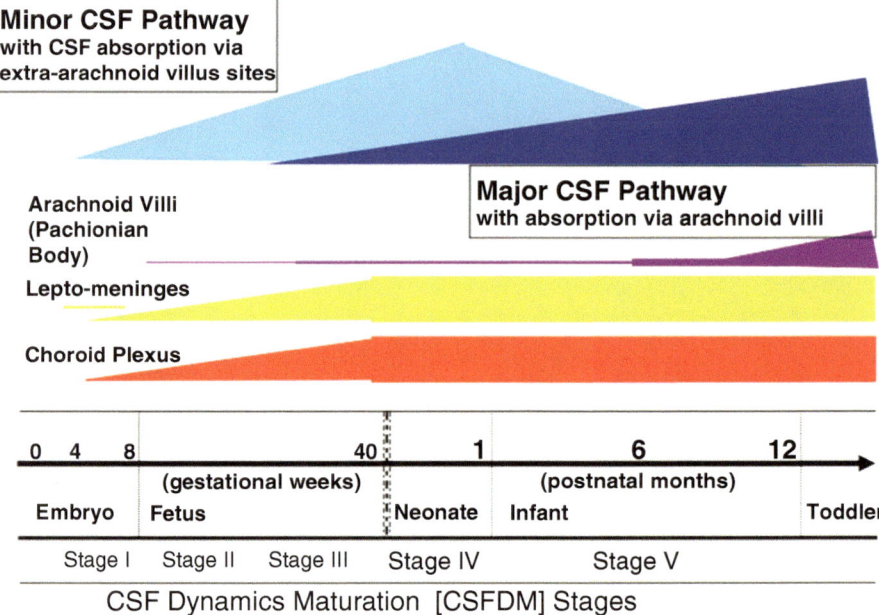

Fig. 2.16 CSF dynamics maturation (CSFDM) stages I–V in the human. (Reprinted from Di Rocco [24]. With permission from Springer Nature)

predominant in the arachnoid granulation, but in the secondary pathway. With age, this mechanism matures through the arachnoid granulation, which becomes increasingly important [24] (Fig. 2.16). Currently, much importance has been attributed to the circulation of cerebrospinal fluid around the blood vessels that penetrate from the subarachnoid space toward the Virchow-Robin space (Fig. 2.17). This space accompanies vessels deep in the cerebral parenchyma and is involved in a significant exchange between cerebrospinal fluid (CSF) and interstitial fluid [23]. This circulation not only serves to cleanse cerebral molecules but also provides interaction with the immune system. During this important exchange, physiological functions may be activated, such as regeneration of the brain during sleep [25]. Currently, regarding the absorption of cerebrospinal fluid (CSF), the importance of aquaporin 4 (AQP4) is also mentioned. It is a membrane transport protein, present in the central nervous system, particularly in the membrane of the astrocytic feet and the basolateral membranes of ependymal cells. It has also been noted that there are no tight junctions between the pia mater and the ependymal cells; thus, water and other substances pass freely between the cerebral parenchyma and subarachnoid space [23].

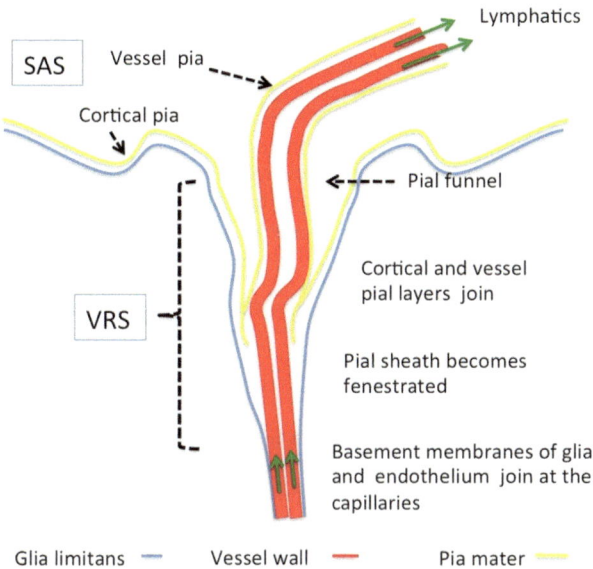

Fig. 2.17 Morphology of the Virchow-Robin space (VRS). Delineated by the basal membranes of the glia, pia, and endothelium, the VRS consists of the space surrounding vessels that penetrate into the parenchyma. The VRS is obliterated at the capillaries where the basement membranes of the glia and endothelium join. The complex pial architecture may be understood as an invagination of both cortical and vessel pia into the VRS. The pial funnel is not a regular finding. The pial sheath around arteries extends into the VRS, but becomes more fenestrated and eventually disappears at the precapillary section of the vessel. Unlike arteries (as shown in this figure), veins do not possess a pial sheath inside the VRS. Interstitial fluid may drain by way of an intramural pathway along the basement membranes of capillaries and arterioles into the lymphatics at the base of the skull (green arrows). It should be noted that the figure does not depict the recently suggested periarterial flow from the subarachnoid space into the parenchyma and an outward flow into the cervical lymphatics along the veins. Also, it is still a matter of debate whether the VRS, extending between the outer basement membrane of the vessel and the glia, represents a fluid-filled open space. Abbreviations: VRS Virchow-Robin space, SAS subarachnoid space. (Reprinted from Brinker et al. [25]. With permission from Creative Commons License 2.0: https://creativecommons.org/licenses/by/2.0/)

References

1. Von Staden H. Herophilus: the art of medicine in early Alexandria. New York: Cambridge University Press; 1989.
2. Mortazavi MM, Adeeb N, Griessenauer CJ, Sheikh H, Shahidi S, Tubbs RI, et al. The ventricular system of the brain: a comprehensive review of its history, anatomy, histology, embryology, and surgical considerations. Childs Nerv Syst. 2014;30:19–35. https://doi.org/10.1007/s00381-013-2321-3.
3. Gross CG. Brain, vision, memory: tales in the history of neuroscience. Cambridge: MIT Press; 1998.

4. Tascioglu AO, Tascioglu AB. Ventricular anatomy: illustrations and concepts from antiquity to renaissance. Neuroanatomy. 2005;4:57–63.
5. Telfer W. Cyril of Jerusalem and Nemesius of Emesa. Philadelphia: Westminster Press; 1955.
6. Corner GW. Anatomical texts of the earlier middle ages: a study in the transmission of cultures. Carnegie Institute of Washington: Washington; 1927.
7. Reisch G. Margarita philosophica. Schott: Freiburg; 1503.
8. Woolam DMH. Concepts of the brain and its functions in classical antiquity. In: Poynter FNL, editor. The history and philosophy of knowledge of the brain and its function. Springfield: Thomas; 1958. p. 48–75.
9. Singer CJ. A short history of anatomy from the Greeks to Harvey. 2nd ed. New York: Dover Publications; 1957.
10. McMurrich JP. Leonardo da Vinci the anatomist. Baltimore: Williams and Wilkins; 1930.
11. Clayton M. Leonardo da Vinci: the anatomy of man. Boston: Little, Brown and Company; 1992.
12. Vinci L, Vangensten OCL, Fonahn A, Hopstock H. Quaderni di anatomia. Jacob Dubwad: Christiania; 1911-1916.
13. Ariès P. The hour of our death. New York: Knopf; 1981.
14. Peccatori S, Zuffi S. Piero della Francesca. London: Dorling Kindersley; 1999.
15. Vesalius A. De humani corporis fabrica libri septem. Johannes Oporinus: Basel; 1543.
16. Santos ARL, Fratzoglou M, Perneczky A. A historical mistake: the aqueduct of Sylvius. Neurosurg Rev. 2004;27:224–5. https://doi.org/10.1007/s10143-004-0334-9.
17. Tubbs RS, Loukas M, Shoja MM, Shokouhi G, Oakes WJ. François Magendie (1783–1855) and his contributions to the foundations of neuroscience and neurosurgery. J Neurosurg. 2008;108:1038–42. https://doi.org/10.3171/JNS/2008/108/5/1038.
18. Von Luschka H. Die Adergeflechte des menschlichen Gehirnes: eine Monographie. Berlin: Georg Reimer; 1855.
19. Key A, Retzius MG. Studien in der Anatomie des Nervensystems und des Bindegewebes. Samson and Wallin: Stockholm; 1875.
20. Dezena RA. Atlas of endoscopic neurosurgery of the third ventricle. Basic principles for ventricular approaches and essential intraoperative anatomy. Cham: Springer International Publishing AG; 2017. https://doi.org/10.1007/978-3-319-50068-3.
21. Rhoton AL Jr. The lateral and third ventricles. Neurosurgery. 2002;51:S207–71.
22. Standring S. Gray's anatomy: the anatomical basis of clinical practice. Edinburgh: Churchill Livingstone; 2008.
23. Miyajima M, Arai H. Evaluation of the production and absorption of cerebrospinal fluid. Neurol Med Chir. 2015;55:647–56. https://doi.org/10.2176/nmc.ra.2015-0003.
24. Oi S, Di Rocco C. Proposal of "evolution theory in cerebrospinal fluid dynamics" and minor pathway hydrocephalus in developing immature brain. Childs Nerv Syst. 2006;22:662–9. https://doi.org/10.1007/s00381-005-0020-4.
25. Brinker T, Stopa E, Morrison J, Klinge P. A new look at cerebrospinal fluid circulation. Fluids Barriers CNS. 2014;11:10. https://doi.org/10.1186/2045-8118-11-10.
26. Hassin GB. The cerebrospinal fluid pathways (a critical note). J Neuropathol Exp Neurol. 1947;6:172–6.
27. Davson H, Segal MB. Physiology of the CSF and blood–brain barriers. 1st ed. New York: CRC Press; 1996.
28. Rodriguez EM, Blazquez JL, Guerra M. The design of barriers in the hypothalamus allows the median eminence and the arcuate nucleus to enjoy private milieus: the former opens to the portal blood and the latter to the cerebrospinal fluid. Peptides. 2010;31:757–76. https://doi.org/10.1016/j.peptides.2010.01.003.
29. Lehtinen MK, Walsh CA. Neurogenesis at the brain–cerebrospinal fluid interface. Annu Rev Cell Dev Biol. 2011;27:653–79. https://doi.org/10.1146/annurevcellbio-092910-154026.
30. Sawamoto K, Wichterle H, Gonzalez-Perez O, Cholfin JA, Yamada M, Spassky N, et al. New neurons follow the flow of cerebrospinal fluid in the adult brain. Science. 2006;311:629–32. https://doi.org/10.1126/science.1119133.

31. Del Bigio MR. The ependyma: a protective barrier between brain and cerebrospinal fluid. Glia. 1995;14:1–13. https://doi.org/10.1002/glia.440140102.

32. Siyahhan B, Knobloch V, de Zélicourt D, Asgari M, Schmid Daners M, Poulikakos D, et al. Flow induced by ependymal cilia dominates near-wall cerebrospinal fluid dynamics in the lateral ventricles. J R Soc Interface. 2014;11:20131189. https://doi.org/10.1098/rsif.2013.1189.

33. Lechtreck KF, Delmotte P, Robinson ML, Sanderson MJ, Witman GB. Mutations in hydin impair ciliary motility in mice. J Cell Biol. 2008;180:633–43. https://doi.org/10.1083/jcb.200710162.

34. Roth Y, Kimhi Y, Edery H, Aharonson E, Priel Z. Ciliary motility in brain ventricular system and trachea of hamsters. Brain Res. 1985;330:291–7. https://doi.org/10.1016/0006-8993(85)90688-2.

35. Ibanez-Tallon I, Pagenstecher A, Fliegauf M, Olbrich H, Kispert A, Ketelsen UP, et al. Dysfunction of axonemal dynein heavy chain Mdnah5 inhibits ependymal flow and reveals a novel mechanism for hydrocephalus formation. Hum Mol Genet. 2004;13:2133–41. https://doi.org/10.1093/hmg/ddh219.

36. Tissir F, Qu Y, Montcouquiol M, Zhou L, Komatsu K, Shi D, et al. Lack of cadherins Celsr2 and Celsr3 impairs ependymal ciliogenesis, leading to fatal hydrocephalus. Nat Neurosci. 2010;13:700–7. https://doi.org/10.1038/nn.2555.

37. Lee L. Riding the wave of ependymal cilia: genetic susceptibility to hydrocephalus in primary ciliary dyskinesia. J Neurosci Res. 2013;91:1117–32. https://doi.org/10.1002/jnr.23238.

38. Davson H. Formation and drainage of the cerebrospinal fluid. Sci Basis Med Annu Rev. 1966:238–59.

39. Davson H, Domer FR, Hollingsworth JR. The mechanism of drainage of the cerebrospinal fluid. Brain. 1973;96:329–36.

40. Johanson CE, Duncan JA 3rd, Klinge PM, Brinker T, Stopa EG, Silverberg GD. Multiplicity of cerebrospinal fluid functions: new challenges in health and disease. Cerebrospinal Fluid Res. 2008;5:10. https://doi.org/10.1186/1743-8454-5-10.

41. Weed LH. Studies on cerebro-spinal fluid. No. II: the theories of drainage of cerebro-spinal fluid with an analysis of the methods of investigation. J Med Res. 1914;31:21–49.

42. Dezena RA. The ventricular system. In: Atlas of endoscopic neurosurgery of the third ventricle. Cham: Springer; 2017. p. 3–34.

Part II
State-of-the-Art

Chapter 3
Endoscopic Ventricular Anatomy

3.1 General Aspects

Between the macroscopic anatomy and the microscopic anatomy, which is also known as histology, there is the mesoscopic anatomy. This term was created by Kurze, and its scale was measured in millimeters [1]. Thus, the mesoscopic anatomy is visualized both in microsurgery and neuroendoscopy. The differentiation between microsurgical and endoscopic anatomy causes difficulties during the performance of endoscopic procedures. One of these differences is that, unlike microsurgery, endoscopy provides a wide angle of view and perspective when it reaches parts that would be optically hidden under the microscope [2, 3], an effect called "fish-eye view." In addition, in endoscopy, the size of the structures changes with the distance of the lenses, and a tiny vessel, when close to the lenses, can be twice the size of the main vessel. The second difference is the requirement of coordination between the hand and eye, in a medium with high need for safety in the direction, orientation, and manipulation of the equipment [2], making the orientation with the use of the endoscope very difficult [2, 4]. It is important to emphasize that microscopic vision yields stereoscopic images, that is, three-dimensional, which neuroendoscopy does not provide, being its main disadvantage. Nowadays 3D monitors can improve the flat visualization. The use of irrigation during endoscopy is an additional element for the production of flat images. Additionally, the geometry of microscopic vision is the opposite of endoscopic vision. While the first corresponds to a pyramid whose apex is at the depth of the operative field and its base is the craniotomy at the surface, the geometry of the endoscopic view is inverted by the optics, thus creating a cone with the apex located at the tip of the neuroendoscope and the base appearing away from it [5]. Microscopic vision allows the surgeon to focus on the depth of field and use, concomitantly, the structures present along the plane of dissection as an anatomical reference [5]. The endoscope lenses are located at the tip of the instrument and provide only the structures located in front of the lenses, but never

© Springer Nature Switzerland AG 2020
R. A. Dezena, *Endoscopic Third Ventriculostomy*,
https://doi.org/10.1007/978-3-030-28657-6_3

along the tube of the instrument [5]. Therefore, while progressing in the depth of the cavity, it is not possible to see the structures left afterwards, unless the endoscope is mobilized. All these factors and limitations give unquestionable importance to the knowledge of the anatomy of the ventricular system [6].

3.2 Lateral Ventricles

Each lateral ventricle is a "C"-shaped cavity that surrounds the thalamus and is deeply located in the brain, following the contour of the choroid fissure. These structures represent, from an embryological point of view, the light of the telencephalic vesicles. Each lateral ventricle has five parts: frontal horn, body, atrium, occipital horn, and temporal horn [7]. The frontal horn is the part of the lateral ventricle located anteriorly to the foramen of Monro. The lateral ventricle body extends from the posterior margin of the foramen of Monro to the point where the fornix and the corpus callosum converge, thus disappearing the septum pellucidum. The atrium of the lateral ventricle and its occipital extension form a triangle with an anterior base in the pulvinar and a posterior apex in the occipital lobe. The occipital horn is triangular, with a posterior vertex and a base in the atrium. The temporal horn is the inferior extension of the ventricle, being the continuation of the atrium, directing itself anteriorly and laterally. Each of these divisions has a medial, lateral, ceiling, and floor wall. In addition, the frontal, temporal, and atrial horns have anterior walls. These walls are formed by the thalamus, septum pellucidum, white matter, corpus callosum, caudate nucleus, and fornix [8, 9]. The foramen of Monro varies from elliptical to circular in shape and communicates the lateral ventricle to the third ventricle. Its path, observed from the ventricular side, is inclined superior and medial and then inferior and lateral [10]. The size and shape of the foramen depend on the size of the ventricles: if the ventricles are small, each foramen is an opening in a crescent shape limited anteriorly by the concave curve of the fornix and posteriorly by the anterior convex tuber of the thalamus. When the ventricles increase in size, the foramen on each side becomes rounder. Its approximate dimensions are 5 × 3 mm [11]. The foramen plane is oriented in such a way that a perpendicular axis is directed medial, ventral, and caudal [12]. The foramen is not only a natural communication between the lateral ventricle and the third ventricle, but it is a region in which structures converge, such as the choroid plexus and important venous structures. The anatomical landmark that seems to be the most reliable for the location of the foramen is the choroid plexus, because the venous structures may be absent, not clearly visible or may vary considerably, in their configuration, in the number of tributaries, or in the place where they enter the choroid fissure to drain into the internal cerebral vein. The most prominent projections of the choroid plexus in the lateral ventricle are located in the temporal horn and in the atrium [11]. In the temporal horn, it spreads laterally, since its fixation in the upper region of the hippocampus. In the atrium, it forms a prominent triangular tuft, called choroid glomus, which can usually be prominent and suggest the presence of a neoplasm in radiological studies. On the margin of the thalamus and fornix, there are small linear depressions, called tenias, in which the choroid plexus is adhered. The tenia on the thalamic side is called the tenia of the thalamus. The tenia on the forniceal side of the fissure is called the tenia of the fornix. The choroidal fissure extends from the foramen of Monro along the medial wall of the central part of the ventricle, atrium and temporal horn, until its inferior termination, the inferior choroidal point, located right after the uncus. The choroid plexus of the third ventricle is projected inferiorly from the roof of the third ventricle on each side of the midline plane. These parallel strips extend from the foramen of Monro to the suprapineal recess and are fixed to the roof of the third ventricle near the medullary stria of the thalamus. The choroid plexuses of the lateral ventricle and the third ventricle are supplied by the anterior choroidal artery and lateral posterior and medial posterior choroidal branches. The anterior choroidal artery originates from the internal carotid artery and enters the temporal horn. The lateral posterior choroidal branches originate from the posterior cerebral artery and enter the temporal horn, atrium, and central part of the lateral ventricle. The medial posterior choroidal branches originate from the posterior cerebral artery and enter the roof of the third ventricle. The intraoperative images demonstrated below have as reference point the Kocher's point, located approximately 2 cm in front of the coronal suture and 2 cm lateral to the midline. This point is the main gateway to the ventricular system for endoscopic procedures [13]. For the lateral ventricle, the endoscopic viewing angle is shown in Figs. 3.1, 3.2, 3.3, and 3.4, followed by images of this region (Figs. 3.5, 3.6, 3.7, and 3.8).

Fig. 3.1 Direction of the endoscopic viewing angle for foramen of Monro region

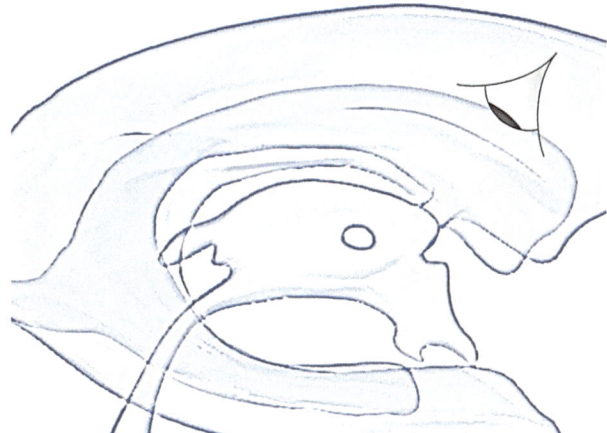

Fig. 3.2 Direction of the endoscopic viewing angle for frontal horn

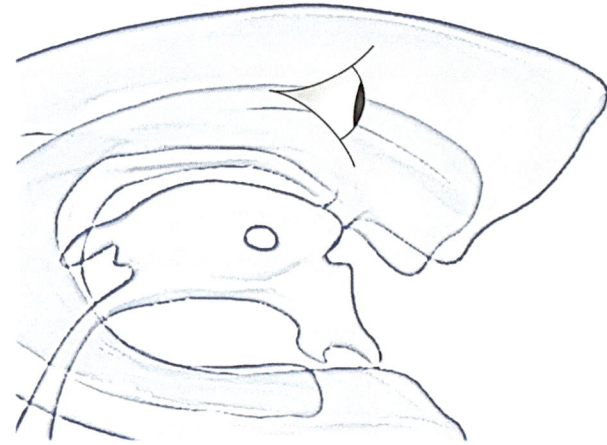

Fig. 3.3 Direction of the endoscopic viewing angle for ventricular body

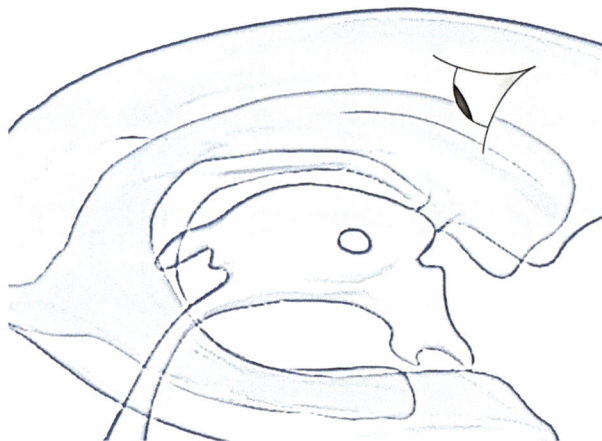

Fig. 3.4 Direction of the endoscopic viewing angle for atrium

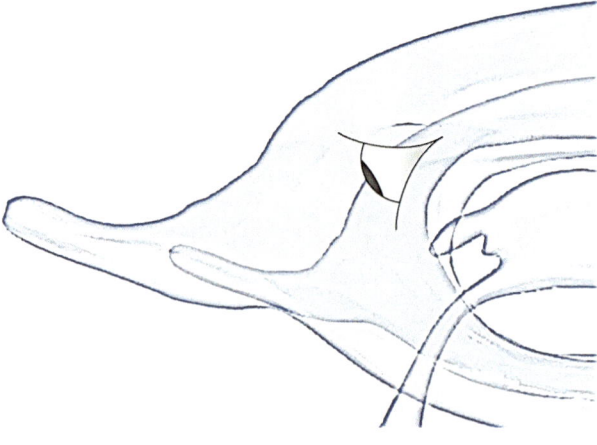

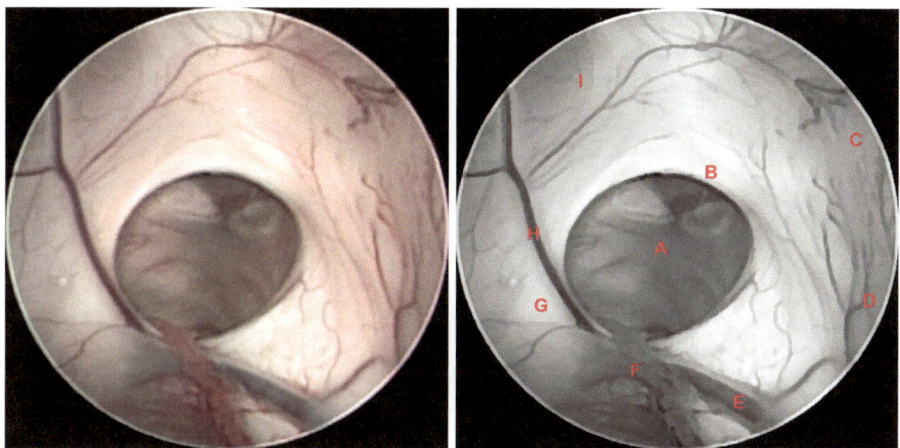

Fig. 3.5 Normal anatomy. (A) Foramen of Monro, (B) column of the fornix, (C) frontal horn, (D) head of the caudate nucleus, (E) superior thalamostriate vein, (F) choroid plexus, (G) body of the fornix, (H) anterior septal vein, (I) septum pellucidum. (Reprinted from Dezena [27]. With permission from Springer Nature)

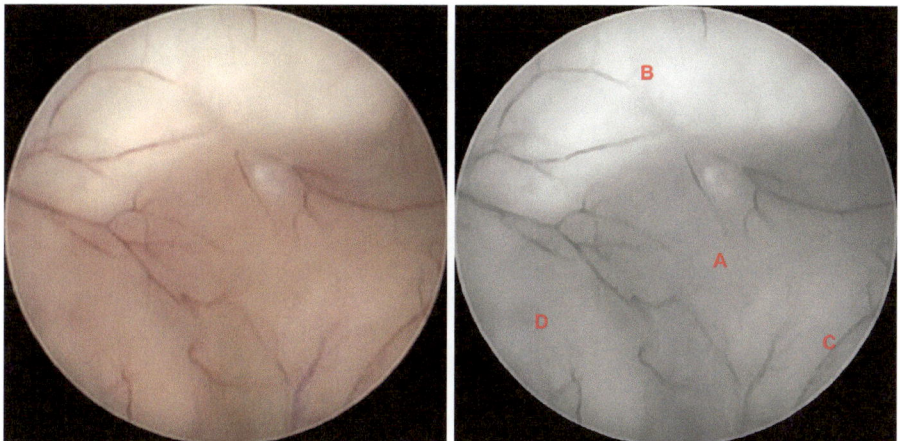

Fig. 3.6 Normal anatomy. (A) Frontal horn, (B) genu of the corpus callosum, (C) head of the caudate nucleus, (D) septum pellucidum. (Reprinted from Dezena [27]. With permission from Springer Nature)

3.3 Third Ventricle

The third ventricle is a funnel-shaped, unilocular, narrow midline cavity. It communicates at the anterosuperior margin with each lateral ventricle through the foramen of Monro and, subsequently, with the fourth ventricle through the cerebral aqueduct. In adult individuals, the lateral distance of the third ventricle is 5.5 mm on average [14]. In a study using MRI images, the hydrocephalic configuration of the third ventricle disappeared after the endoscopic third ventriculostomy (ETV), with a decrease in diameter, elevation, and horizontal direction of the floor and

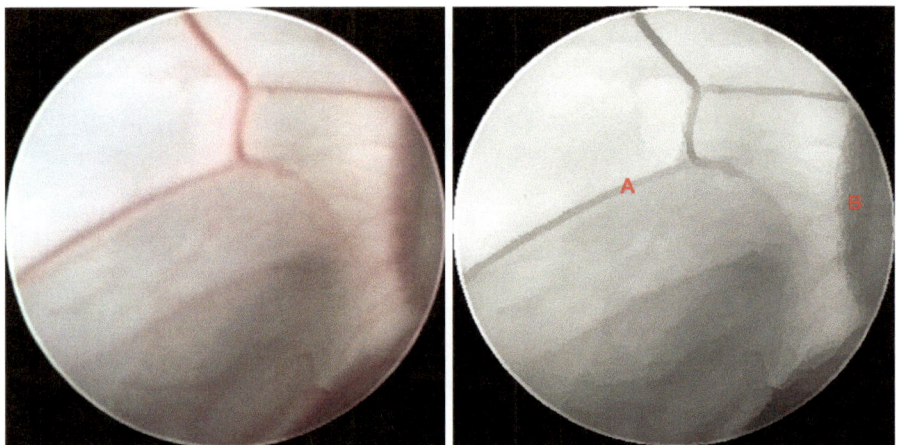

Fig. 3.7 Normal anatomy. (A) Septal veins, (B) anterior septal vein. (Reprinted from Dezena [27]. With permission from Springer Nature)

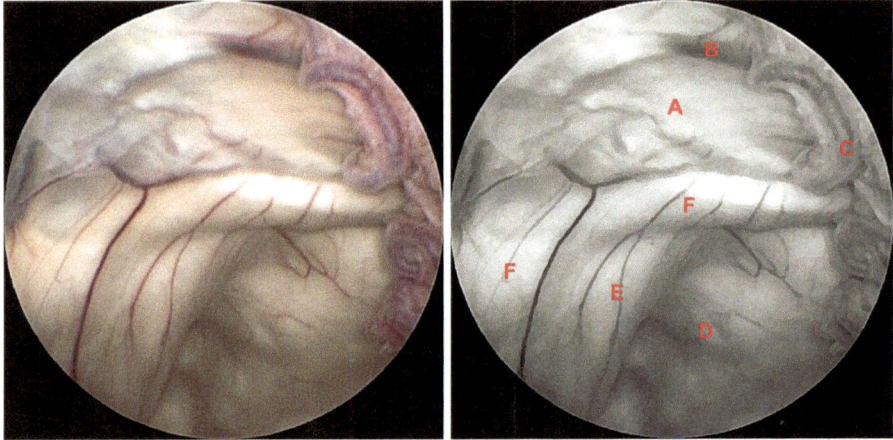

Fig. 3.8 Normal anatomy. (A) Septum pellucidum, (B) posterior septal vein, (C) superior choroidal vein, (D) collateral eminence, (E) calcar avis, (F) bulb of the occipital horn. (Reprinted from Dezena [27]. With permission from Springer Nature)

reduction of the infundibular angle [15]. The floor of the third ventricle extends from the optic chiasm anteriorly to the opening of the cerebral aqueduct posteriorly. It descends ventral and is formed by at least 12 cellular clusters or nuclei within the hypothalamic region [16]. Anatomically, three portions can be described on the floor of the third ventricle: (1) premammillary portion, which extends from the infundibulum to the premammillary sulcus, constituting a very thin layer of gray substance of the hypothalamus; (2) interpeduncular portion, which extends from the postmammillary recess to the posterior margin of the interpeduncular space, being formed of gray substance and firmer than the first; and (3) peduncular portion, which corresponds to the portion of the cerebral peduncles, being the most solid portion, being formed by the medial aspect of the peduncles covered by the peduncular ependyma. This portion normally forms a very soft angle with the interpeduncular portion, thus facilitating the recognition of its anterior limit [17]. The anterior half of the floor is formed by the diencephalic structures and the posterior half by the mesencephalic structures. When visualized by the inferior part, the structures that form the floor include from anterior to posterior: optic chiasm, infundibulum, tuber cinereum, mammillary bodies, posterior perforated substance, and part of the tegmentum of the mesencephalon located superior to the medial aspect of the cerebral peduncles. The infundibulum is a hollow, funnel-shaped structure located between the optical chiasm and the tuber cinereum, with a reddish-yellow color, which corresponds to the implantation of the pituitary stalk on the floor [5]. The pituitary gland is connected to the infundibulum, and the axons of the infundibulum extend to the posterior part of the pituitary gland. When the third ventricle is observed superior and internally, the optical chiasm forms a transverse eminence in the anterior margin of the floor [12, 18]. The recess of the infundibulum extends into the infundibulum posterior to the optic chiasm, a slightly orange or reddish area [19]. The part of the floor between the mammillary bodies and the cerebral aqueduct presents a smooth surface that is concave from one side to the other. This surface covers the posterior perforated substance, anteriorly, and part of the medial of the cerebral peduncles and tegmentum of the mesencephalon, posteriorly. The most important anatomical references on the floor for the ETV are the mammillary bodies and the infundibulum as well as the pulsating basilar artery [20]. As long as the distance between the mammillary bodies and infundibulum is 6 mm, there is ample space for a safe ETV [21]. In hydrocephalic patients, the floor of the third ventricle can be elevated to the level of the infundibulum recess compared to the mammillary bodies, and for this reason, the puncture of the floor of the third ventricle can be difficult [19]. The tuber cinereum is a prominent mass of hypothalamic gray substance located before the mammary bodies, which merges anteriorly with the infundibulum. The region of the tuber cinereum around the base of the infundibulum is elevated, forming a prominence called median eminence of the hypothalamus. Laterally, the tuber cinereum is delimited by the optical tracts and cerebral peduncles [22]. When visualized by the endoscope from the third ventricle, the tuber cinereum is translucent and dark blue, while the recess of the infundibulum is light red. The tuber cinereum is demonstrable not only posteriorly but also anteriorly to the optic chiasm [23]. The blood irrigation of the tuber cinereum originates from the inferior diencephalic branches in number from one to ten, mainly from the posterior communicating artery [24] and the internal carotid artery [23, 25]. The mammillary bodies form round prominences, posteriorly to the tuber cinereum. In the hypothalamus, the mammillary bodies are the only nuclei identified on the MRI image [16]. They are spherical structures, approximately 5 mm in diameter, located lower in the brain, at the posterior limit of the hypothalamus. They are composed of two nuclei, one more prominent medial and one lateral [26]. In endoscopic terms, the third ventricle can be divided into anterior, middle, and posterior segments [13] (Fig. 3.9).

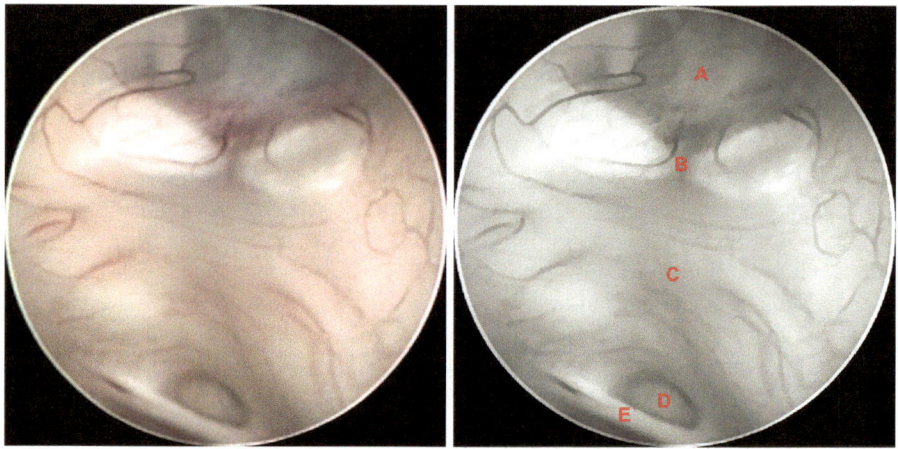

Fig. 3.9 Normal anatomy. (A) Tuber cinereum, (B) mammillary bodies, (C) middle segment, (D) cerebral aqueduct, (E) posterior commissure. (Reprinted from Dezena [28]. With permission from Springer Nature)

Fig. 3.10 Direction of the endoscopic viewing angle for the anterior segment of the third ventricle

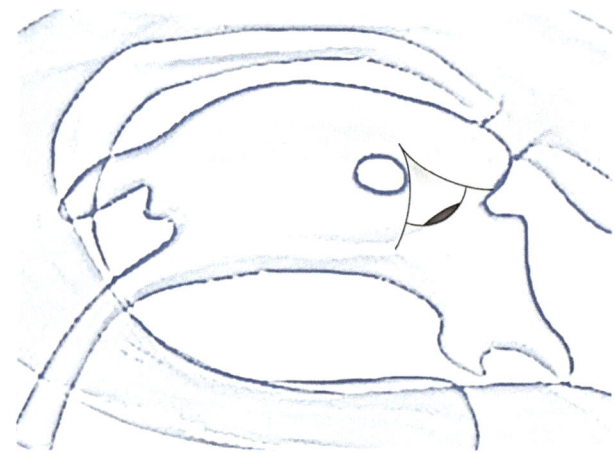

3.3.1 Anterior Segment

The knowledge of the endoscopic anatomy of the anterior segment of the third ventricle is of paramount importance for the performance of endoscopic third ventriculostomy. For the anterior segment, the endoscopic viewing angle is shown in Fig. 3.10, followed by the image of this region (Fig. 3.11).

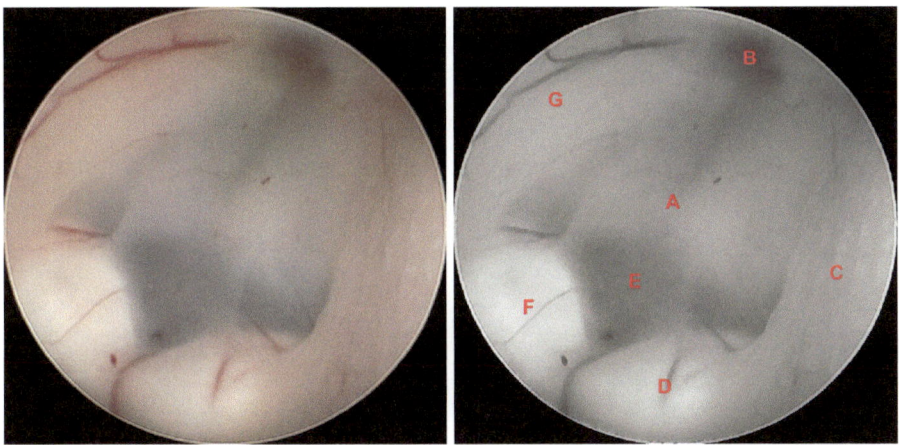

Fig. 3.11 Normal anatomy. (A) Tuber cinereum, (B) infundibular recess, (C) right hypothalamus, (D) right mammillary body, (E) premammillary recess, (F) left mammillary body, (G) left hypothalamus. (Reprinted from Dezena [28]. With permission from Springer Nature)

Fig. 3.12 Direction of the endoscopic viewing angle for the middle segment of the third ventricle

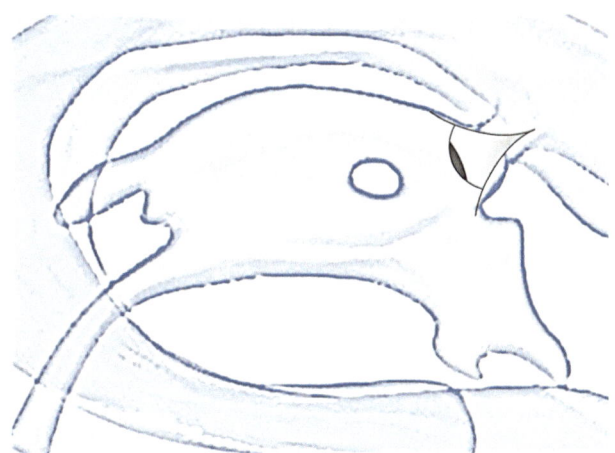

3.3.2   Middle Segment

The middle segment usually presents the interthalamic adhesion, which may be more or less prominent depending on the patient's age, and is more present in children. For the middle segment, the endoscopic viewing angle is shown in Fig. 3.12, followed by the image of this region (Fig. 3.13).

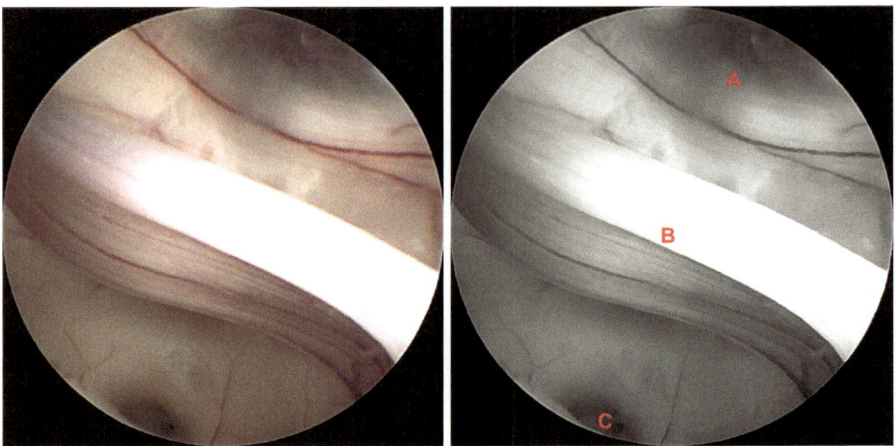

Fig. 3.13 Normal anatomy. (A) Postmammillary recess, (B) interthalamic adhesion, (C) cerebral aqueduct entrance. (Reprinted from Dezena [28]. With permission from Springer Nature)

Fig. 3.14 Direction of the endoscopic viewing angle for the posterior segment of the third ventricle

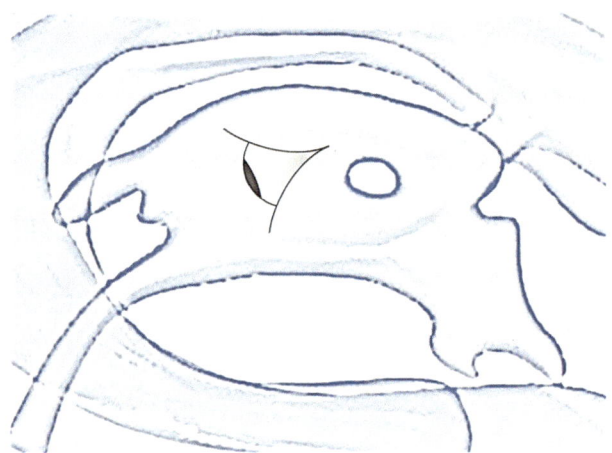

3.3.3   Posterior Segment

Knowledge of the anatomy of the posterior segment is useful for endoscopic procedures such as aqueductoplasty and tumor biopsies. For the posterior segment, the endoscopic viewing angle is shown in Fig. 3.14, followed by images of this region (Fig. 3.15).

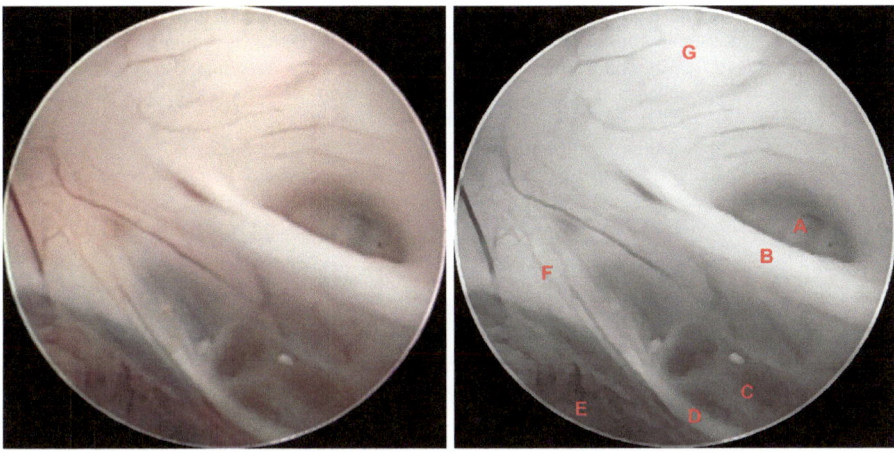

Fig. 3.15 Normal anatomy. (A) Cerebral aqueduct entrance, (B) posterior commissure, (C) pineal recess and pineal gland, (D) habenular commissure, (E) suprapineal recess, (F) habenular trigone, (G) left thalamus. (Reprinted from Dezena [28]. With permission from Springer Nature)

References

1. Jannetta PJ. Gross (mesoscopic) description of the human trigeminal nerve and ganglion. J Neurosurg. 1967;26(1):109–11.
2. Resch KD, Perneczky A, Tschabitscher M, Kindel S. Endoscopic anatomy of the ventricles. Acta Neurochir Suppl. 1994;61:57–61.
3. Burtscher J, Dessl A, Maurer H, Seiwald M, Felber S. Virtual neuroendoscopy, a comparative magnetic resonance and anatomical study. Minim Invasive Neurosurg. 1999;42(3):113–7.
4. Matula C, Tschabitscher M, Kitz K, Reinprecht A, Koos WT. Neuroanatomical details under endoscopical view- relevant for radiosurgery? Acta Neurochir Suppl. 1995;63:1–4.
5. King WA, Frazee JG, De Salles AAF. Endoscopy of the central and peripheral nervous system. New York: Thieme; 1998.
6. Romero ADCB, Aguiar PHP, Borchartt TB, Conci A. Quantitative ventricular neuroendoscopy performed on the third ventriculostomy: anatomic study. Neurosurgery. 2011;68(2 Suppl Operative):347–54; discussion 353–4. https://doi.org/10.1227/NEU.0b013e318211449a.
7. Jacobson S, Marcus EM. Meninges, ventricular system and vascular system. In: Jacobson S, Marcus EM, editors. Neuroanatomy for the neuroscientist. New York: Springer; 2008. p. 399–407.
8. Rhoton AL. The lateral and third ventricles. Neurosurgery. 2002;51(suppl 1):209–72.
9. Timurkaynak E, Rhoton AL, Barry M. Microsurgical anatomy and operative approaches to the lateral ventricles. Neurosurgery. 1986;19(5):685–723.
10. Grunert P, Perneczky A, Resch KDM. Endoscopic procedures through the foramen interventriculare of Monro under stereotactical conditions. Minim Invasive Neurosurg. 1994;37(1):2–8.
11. Fujii K, Lenkey C, Rhoton AL. Microsurgical anatomy of the choroidal arteries: lateral and third ventricles. J Neurosurg. 1980;52(2):165–88.

12. Cuello LM, Gagliardi CE. Anatomía endoscópica del sistema ventricular. In: Técnicas actuales en neurocirugía endoscópica. Buenos Aires: Ediciones de la Guadalupe; 2007. p. 95–106.
13. Dezena RA. Atlas of endoscopic neurosurgery of the third ventricle. Basic principles for ventricular approaches and essential intraoperative anatomy. Cham: Springer International Publishing AG; 2017. https://doi.org/10.1007/978-3-319-50068-3.
14. Lang J. Anatomy of the midline. Acta Neurochir Suppl. 1985;35:6–22.
15. Ernestus R-I, Krüger K, Ernst S, Lackner K, Klug N. Relevance of magnetic resonance imaging for ventricular endoscopy. Minim Invasive Neurosurg. 2002;45(2):72–7.
16. Loes DJ, Barloon TJ, Yuh WT, DeLaPaz RL, Sato Y. MR anatomy and pathology of the hypothalamus. AJR Am J Roentgenol. 1991;156(3):579–85.
17. Corrales M, Torrealba G. The third ventricle. Normal anatomy and changes in some pathological conditions. Neuroradiology. 1976;11(5):271–7.
18. Vinas FC, Dujovny N, Dujovny M. Microanatomical basis for the third ventriculostomy. Minim Invasive Neurosurg. 1996;39(4):116–21.
19. Çataltepe O. Endoscopic third ventriculostomy: indications, surgical technique, and potential problems. Turk Neurosurg. 2002;12:65–73.
20. Zohdi A, Ibrahim I. Variations in the site and size of third ventriculocisternostomy. Minim Invasive Neurosurg. 1998;41(4):194–7.
21. Lang J. Topographic anatomy of preformed intracranial spaces. Acta Neurochir Suppl. 1992;54:1–10.
22. Oka K, Go Y, Kin Y, Tomonaga M. An observation of the third ventricle under flexible fiber optic ventriculoscope: normal structure. Surg Neurol. 1993;40(4):273–7.
23. Lang J. Surgical anatomy of the hypothalamus. Acta Neurochir. 1985;75(1–4):5–22.
24. Vinas FC, Panigrahi M. Microsurgical anatomy of the Liliequist membrane and surrounding neurovascular territories. Minim Invasive Neurosurg. 2001;44(2):104–9.
25. Romero ADCB, Silva CE, Aguiar PHP. The distance between the posterior communicating arteries and their relation to the endoscopic third ventriculostomy in adults: an anatomic study. Surg Neurol Int. 2011;2:91. https://doi.org/10.4103/2152-7806.82373.
26. Denby CE, Vann SD, Tsivilis D, Aggleton JP, Montaldi D, Roberts N, Mayes AR. The frequency and extent of mammillary body atrophy associated with surgical removal of a colloid cyst. Am J Neuroradiol. 2009;30(4):736–43. https://doi.org/10.3174/ajnr.A1424.
27. Dezena RA. Entering the third ventricle: the lateral ventricle. In: Atlas of endoscopic neurosurgery of the third ventricle. Cham: Springer; 2017. p. 69–119.
28. Dezena RA. Inside the third ventricle. In: Atlas of endoscopic neurosurgery of the third ventricle. Cham: Springer; 2017. p. 121–208.

Chapter 4
Basic Principles of Endoscopic Neurosurgery

4.1 General Concepts

Neuroendoscopy has been widely disseminated in the last two decades, mainly due to the development of modern optical systems, cameras, and HD monitors. Based on these advances, the technique was consolidated and definitively integrated with the arsenal of global neurosurgical techniques. Currently, it is mandatory that neuroendoscopy be integrated with the neurosurgical training of residents. The neurosurgeon who was not trained in the technique during residency is offered hands-on courses of the highest quality worldwide. Currently, cerebral endoscopy can be classified under endoscopic neurosurgery, endoscope-controlled microneurosurgery, and endoscope-assisted microneurosurgery [1–3]. Examples of the latter two, respectively, are endonasal surgeries for pituitary tumors and endoscopic intraoperative inspection of microsurgical clipping of cerebral aneurysms. Endoscopic neurosurgery or "channel endoscopy" consists of the use of neuroendoscopic optics in the ventricular cavity, with the instruments being used through one or more of the neuroendoscopy system's work channels. It is important to remember that, when compared to the surgical microscope, the endoscope provides a completely different view, with advantages and disadvantages. Current systems of ventricular neuroendoscopy with the Hopkins rod-lens system (Karl Storz GmbH & Co. KG, Tuttlingen, Germany) (Fig. 4.1), the most widely used in the world, provide excellent image resolution and good panoramic (wide-angle) vision, and even lesions not located directly in front of the endoscope can be visualized [1, 2]. Through this panoramic view, ventricular navigation is judged to be extremely accurate and safe. Another major advantage of the neuroendoscope is that there is no need to adjust the focus during the procedure, unlike the surgical microscope, where continuous adjustment is necessary, especially at high magnifications. On the other hand, the most obvious disadvantage of the neuroendoscope is the lack of stereoscopic vision. This deficiency is mitigated by a phenomenon derived from astronomy, known as parallax. This phenomenon consists of the perception that objects closer to the neuroendoscope move more when compared to

© Springer Nature Switzerland AG 2020
R. A. Dezena, *Endoscopic Third Ventriculostomy*,
https://doi.org/10.1007/978-3-030-28657-6_4

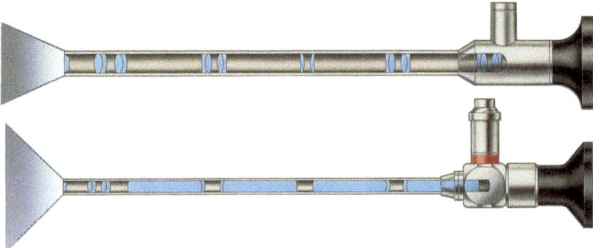

Fig. 4.1 Hopkins rod-lens system. [© KARL STORZ SE & Co. KG, Germany]

the more distant objects, providing a pseudo 3D effect [1, 2]. The lack of stereoscopic vision is compensated by experimental training and the learning curve. Another major drawback is the lower image resolution when compared to the microscope. This is due to the microscope's own characteristics, such as larger diameter objective lenses, and the fact that the surgeon is looking directly at the structures through the lens system, with the retina being the sensor that captures the image. In the endoscope, the sensor that captures the image is the CCD, located in the head of the camera and coupled to the optics. Even with the recent introduction of full HD cameras, with extremely high resolution, which produces images of 1080 lines and 2 million pixels, this image is still not comparable to the power of the human retina [2]. General indications for endoscopic neurosurgery are obstructions in cerebrospinal fluid flow, ventricular and paraventricular arachnoid cysts, and intraventricular lesions [4–7]. The most common techniques to restore cerebrospinal fluid circulation are endoscopic third ventriculostomy, septostomy, foraminoplasty, aqueductoplasty with or without stents, cystic fenestrations, and biopsies and tumor resections [8–14].

4.2 Basic Techniques

The most common point for access to the ventricular system is Kocher's point, which is approximately 2 cm anterior to the coronal suture and 2 cm lateral to the midline (Fig. 4.2). Other ventricular access points may be used depending on the disease to be treated [15] (Fig. 4.3). In adults and children older than 1 year, the opening in the skull can be performed through a drill hole, and in infants the fontanelle may be a physiological corridor to the neuroendoscope [16] (Figs. 4.4 and 4.5). Before starting the surgery, it is important to check the position of the monitor so that it is as comfortable as possible for the surgeon. Ideally, the monitor should be placed at the level of the surgeon's eyes and immediately in front of him, to avoid synkinesis movements of the arms concomitant with the movement of the eyes. In adults and older children, the skull perforation can be performed with a high-rotation motor, and the dura mater opening is performed in cross with bipolar coagulation of its edges. In newborns, the dura mater is opened in linear format to allow its closure after surgery [16] (Fig. 4.6). In endoscopic neurosurgery, the neuroendoscope itself

Fig. 4.2 Kocher's point in an adult

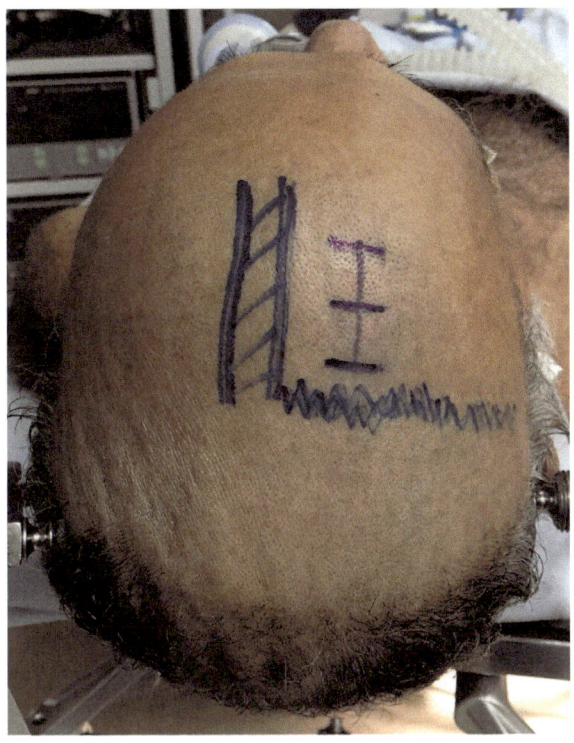

Fig. 4.3 Schematic illustration of all the extra-calvarial ventricular access points: Keen (1), Kocher (2), Dandy (3), Frazier (4), Kaufman (5), and Tubbs (6). (Reprinted from Mortazavi et al. [15]. With permission from Springer Nature)

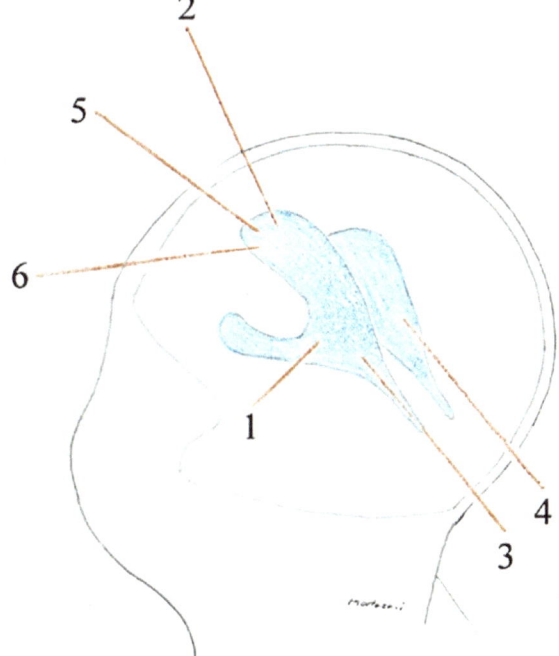

Fig. 4.4 3D CT scan depicting the burr hole at Kocher's point in an adult

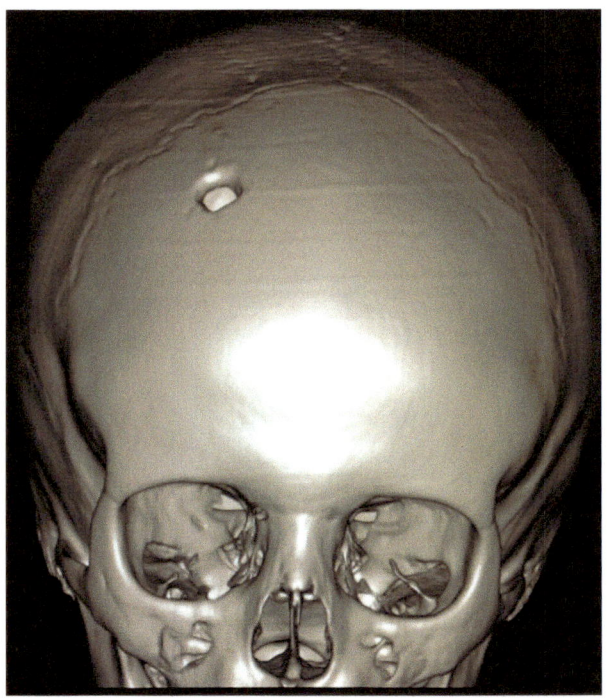

Fig. 4.5 Detail of the transfontanelle approach

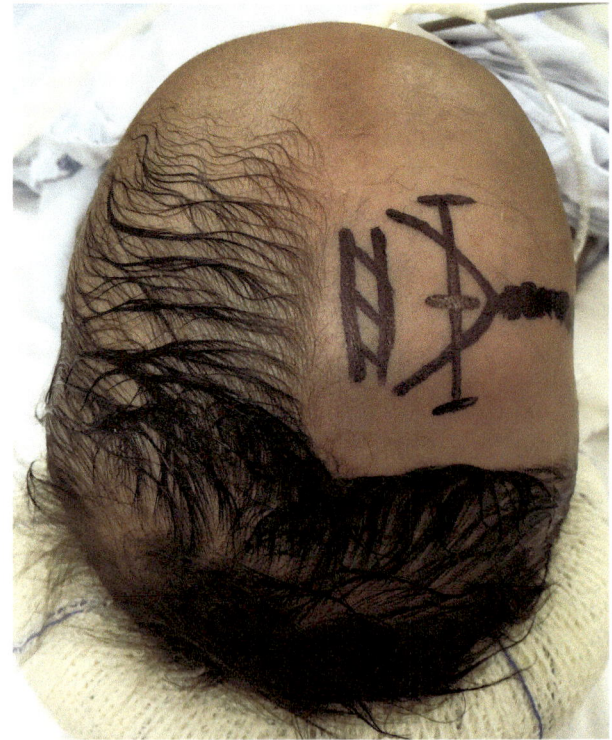

is the visualization tool and through which the instruments travel through the working channels of each system. Currently, several systems are available in the market, each with advantages and disadvantages. Compact systems such as the Oi HandyPro and Gaab systems (Karl Storz GmbH & Co. KG, Tuttlingen, Germany) allow free-hand movements in addition to excellent image quality (Figs. 4.7 and 4.8). After ventricular puncture, it is possible to perform four-handed surgery, with the help of

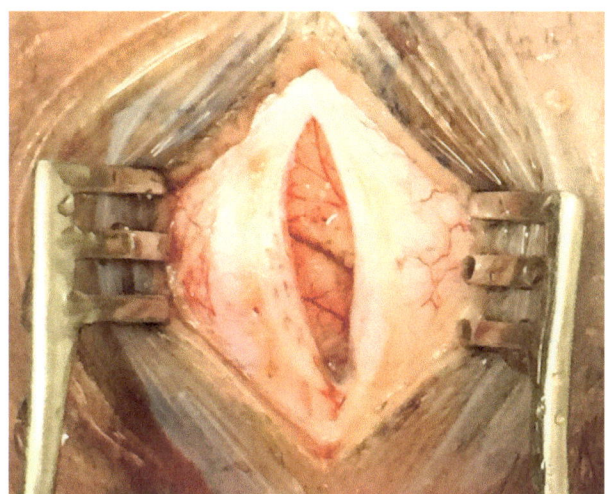

Fig. 4.6 Dural opening in a linear fashion in a newborn. (Reprinted from Dezena [21]. With permission from Springer Nature)

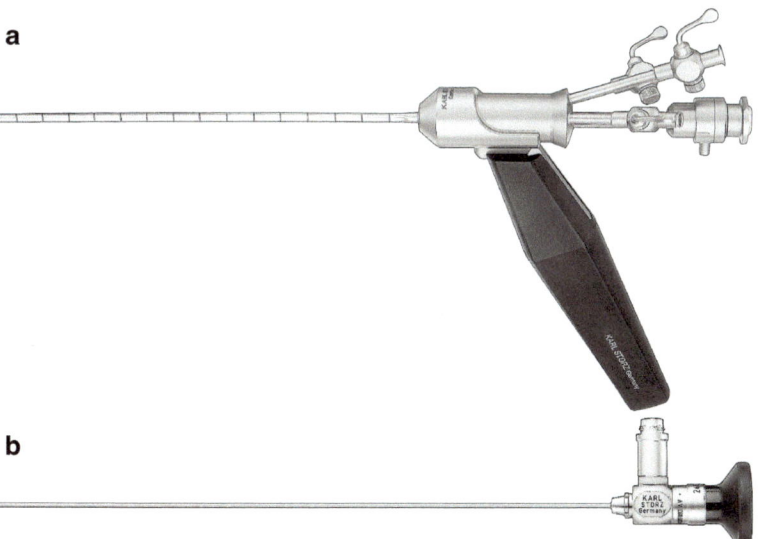

Fig. 4.7 Oi HandyPro system, with removable handle, including operating sheath handle (3 work channel) and mandrel (**a**), and wide-angle straight forward telescope 0° (enlarged view, diameter 2 mm, length 26 cm) (**b**). Instruments (diameter 1.3 mm, working length 30 cm) including scissors (single action jaws), biopsy forceps (double action jaws), grasping forceps (double action jaws), unipolar coagulation electrode, and bipolar coagulation electrode (**c**). [© KARL STORZ SE & Co. KG, Germany]

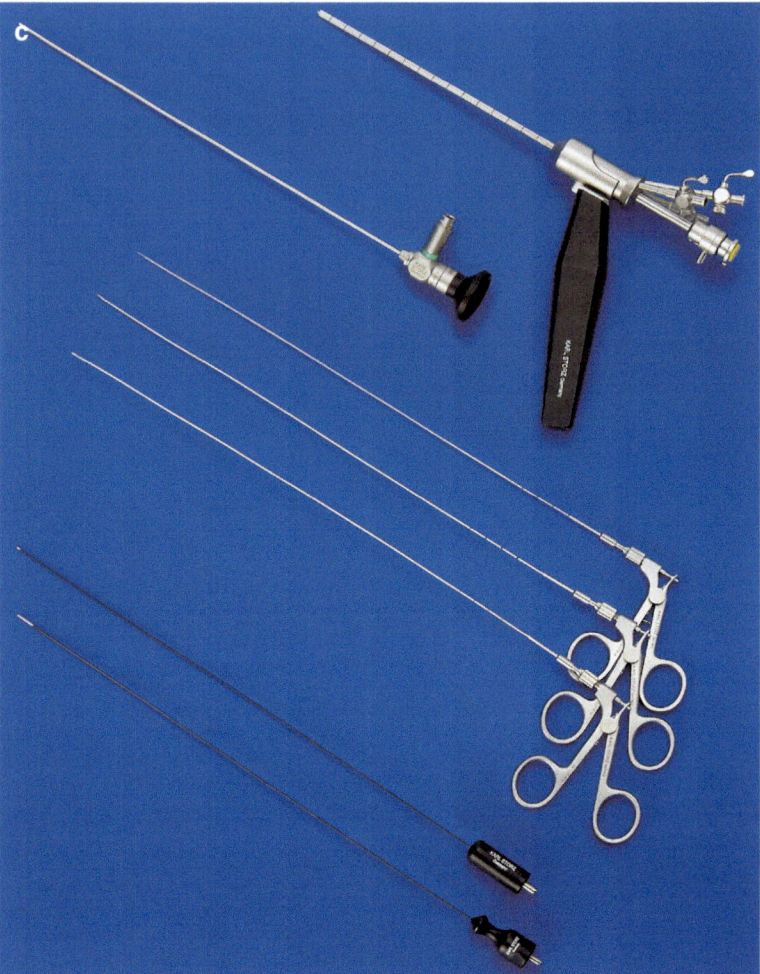

Fig. 4.7 (continued)

Fig. 4.8 Gaab system, including telescope with wide-angle straight forward telescope 6°, with working channel diameter 3 mm, length 15 cm and operating sheath, graduated, outer diameter 6.5 mm, working length 13 cm, with lateral stopcock and catheter port and obturator (**a**). Instruments including grasping forceps (single action jaws, diameter 2.7 mm, working length 30 cm), biopsy forceps (single action jaws, diameter 2.7 mm, working length 30 cm), scissors (pointed, single action jaws, diameter 2.7 mm, working length 30 cm), scissors (pointed, slightly curved, double action jaws, diameter 1.7 mm, working length 30 cm), biopsy forceps (double action jaws, diameter 1.7 mm, working length 30 cm), forceps for ventriculostomy (diameter 1.7 mm, working length 30 cm), bipolar forceps (with flat jaws, size 2.4 mm, working length 24 cm), bipolar coagulation electrode (diameter 1.7 mm, working length 30 cm), unipolar coagulation electrode (semiflexible, diameter 1.7 mm, working length 30 cm), suction catheter (flexible, for single use, diameter 2.5 mm, working length 45 cm), irrigation tube, and holding system (**b**). [© KARL STORZ SE & Co. KG, Germany]

an assistant, or freehand. Some neuroendoscopists prefer an articulated support to keep the neuroendoscope fixed and allow the surgeon to keep both hands free to manipulate the instruments through the work channels, depending on the neuroendoscopy type. Another alternative is that a neuroendoscopist manipulates the optics and the assistant handles the instruments without worrying about navigation [17]. In

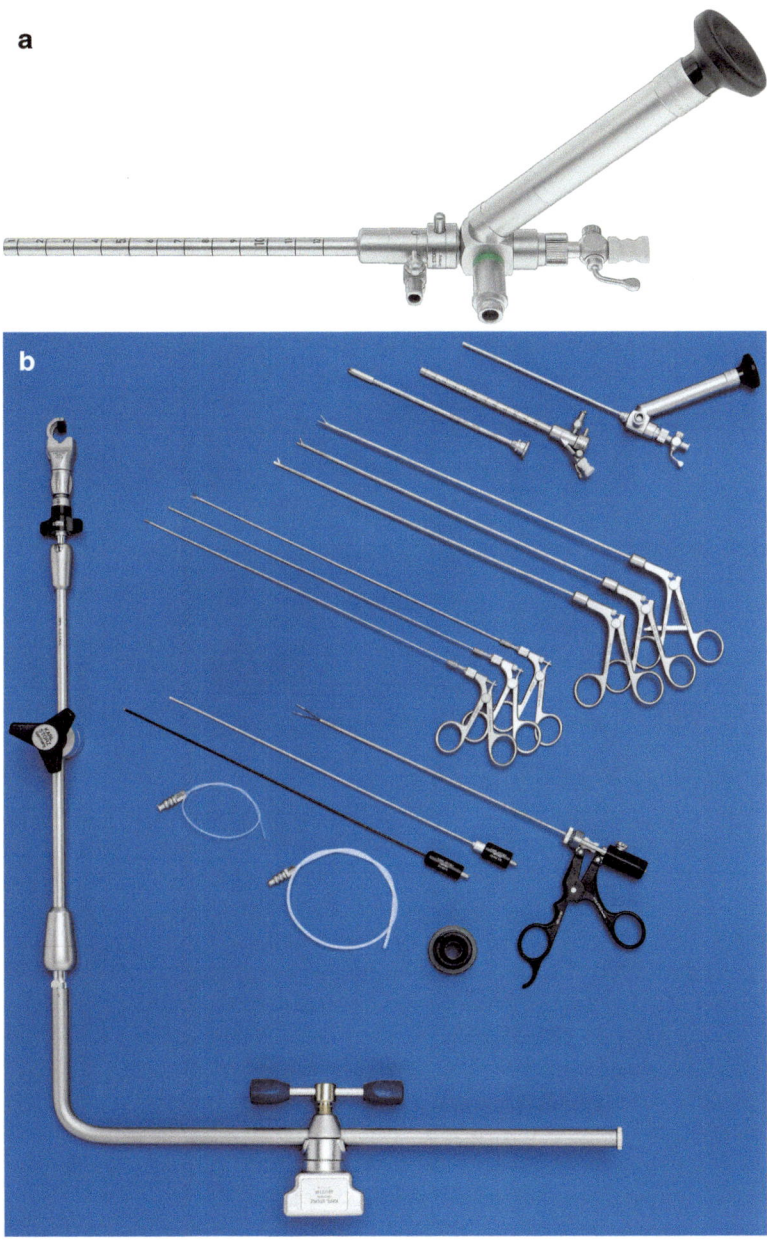

Fig. 4.9 Oi HandyPro
frameless freehand system
in action

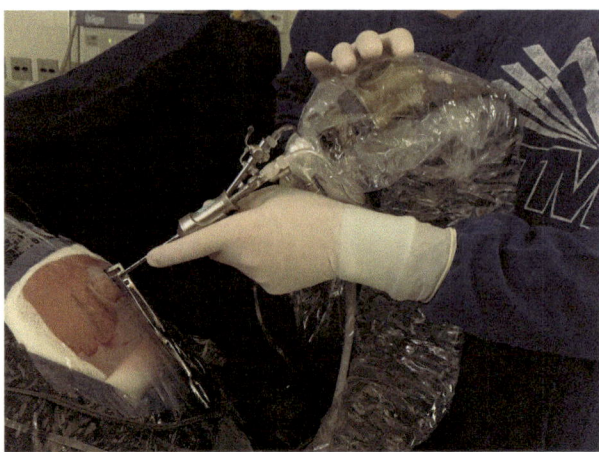

Fig. 4.10 Freehand
technique by Gaab system,
holding neuroendoscope with
non-dominant hand and
handle instrument (scissors)
with dominant hand

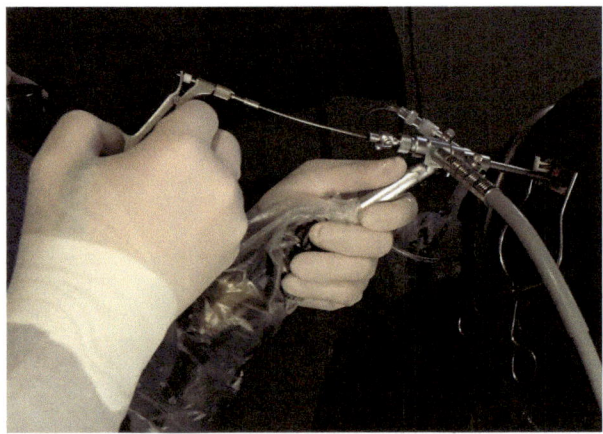

this case, in some systems with more than one working channel, there is possibility
of some manual dissection, coaxially, obviously not as elegant as in the surgical
microscope [18]. A third alternative, which is undoubtedly the best, since it allows
the completely unhindered movement of the endoscope, is the freehand technique
[19]. In this mode, by a unique neuroendoscopist, the navigation or handling of the
optics is performed with the non-dominant hand, and the manipulation of the instruments is performed with the dominant hand. The Oi system is specially designed for
this purpose [19, 20] (Fig. 4.9). The Gaab system, although not designed specifically for this technique, is suitable for this, given its compact profile (Fig. 4.10).
Since endoscopic navigation occurs in a clear, liquid medium, even a minimal
amount of blood could render visualization of structures impossible. Because of
this, continuous irrigation with saline or Ringer lactate solution, always heated to
body temperature, through the neuroendoscopy system is mandatory, which also
contributes to prevent ventricular collapse. It is possible for the neuroendoscopist to

perform the procedures sitting or standing depending on the duration of the surgery. After the completion of the endoscopic time, the correct closure is of extreme importance. In adults and older children, Gelfoam is used in the cortical/subcortical tunnel, which has the function of containing the biological glue that will be used on this. The scalp is closed by layers at separate points using absorbable suture threads (Vicryl) in the aponeurosis and nonabsorbable suture threads (mononylon) on the skin [16]. On the other hand, in newborns Gelfoam is not used because the layer of cortex is thin. The dural closure is performed with nonabsorbable suture threads (polypropylene or silk) and placement of biological glue over the suture. The scalp is closed by layers at separate points using absorbable suture threads (Vicryl) in the aponeurosis and nonabsorbable threads (mononylon) on the skin [16] (Figs. 4.11 and 4.12). The recording and archiving of the videos of each procedure have

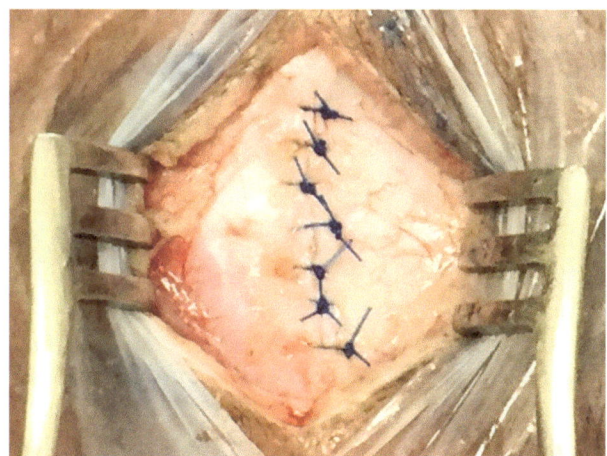

Fig. 4.11 Polypropylene dural watertight closure. Silk or cotton suture can be good options. (Reprinted from Dezena [21]. With permission from Springer Nature)

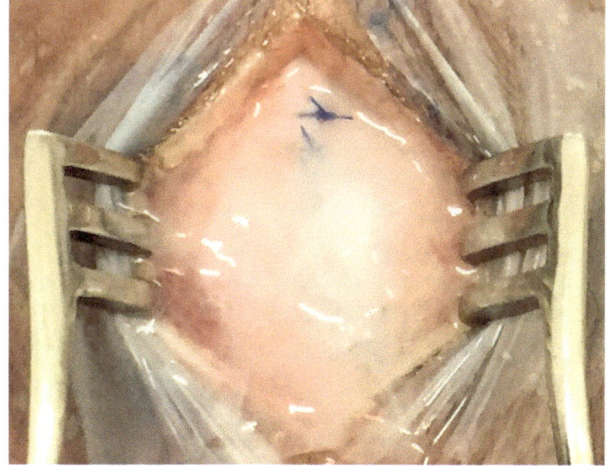

Fig. 4.12 Biological glue over suture. (Reprinted from Dezena [21]. With permission from Springer Nature)

Fig. 4.13 AIDA system. A solution for the recording of patient data, full HD videos, and images. [© KARL STORZ SE & Co. KG, Germany]

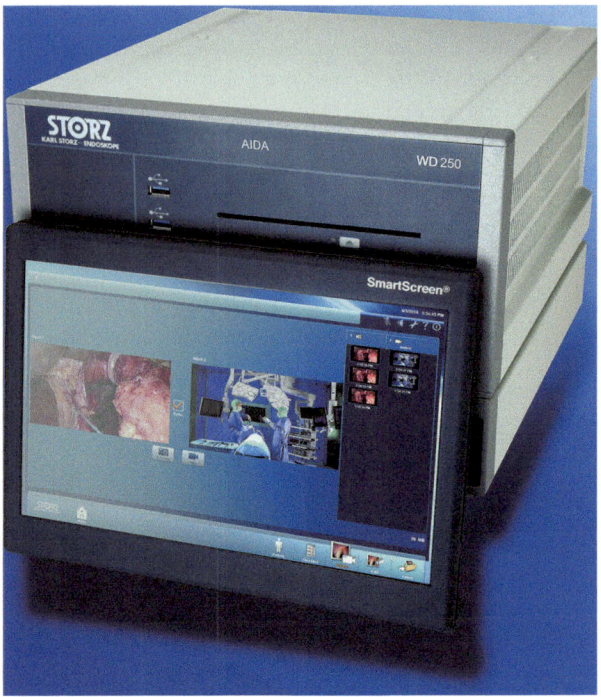

scientific importance for educational, training, and publication purposes, as well as having a legal role. The AIDA system (Karl Storz GmbH & Co. KG, Tuttlingen, Germany) offers a solution for the recording of patient data and full HD videos and still images. An intuitive interface and user-friendly front panel supports fast and uncomplicated handling (Fig. 4.13).

References

1. Schroeder HWS. Current status and future developments of neuroendoscopically assisted neurosurgery. In: Sgouros S, editor. Neuroendoscopy. Berlin/Heidelberg: Springer; 2014. p. 65–80. https://doi.org/10.1007/978-3-642-39085-2_6.
2. Schroeder HW, Nehlsen M. Value of high-definition imaging in neuroendoscopy. Neurosurg Rev. 2009;32:303–8. https://doi.org/10.1007/s10143-009-0200-x.
3. Hopf NJ, Perneczky A. Endoscopic neurosurgery and endoscope-assisted microneurosurgery for the treatment of intracranial cysts. Neurosurgery. 1998;43:1330–6.
4. Gaab MR, Schroeder HW. Neuroendoscopic approach to intraventricular lesions. Neurosurg Focus. 1999;6:e5.
5. Schroeder HW, Gaab MR. Endoscopic resection of colloid cysts. Neurosurgery. 2002;51:1441–4.
6. Schroeder HW, Gaab MR, Niendorf WR. Indications for endoscopic neurosurgery in children. Childs Nerv Syst. 1996;12:485–6.

7. Schroeder HW, Gaab MR, Niendorf WR. Neuroendoscopic approach to arachnoid cysts. J Neurosurg. 1996;85:293–8. https://doi.org/10.3171/jns.1996.85.2.0293.
8. Gaab MR, Schroeder HW. Neuroendoscopic approach to intraventricular lesions. J Neurosurg. 1998;88:496–505. https://doi.org/10.3171/jns.1998.88.3.0496.
9. Oertel JM, Baldauf J, Schroeder HW, Gaab MR. Endoscopic options in children: experience with 134 procedures. J Neurosurg Pediatr. 2009;3:81–9. https://doi.org/10.3171/2008.11.PEDS0887.
10. Oertel JM, Schroeder HW, Gaab MR. Endoscopic stomy of the septum pellucidum: indications, technique, and results. Neurosurgery. 2009;64:482–91. https://doi.org/10.1227/01.NEU.0000338944.42411.67.
11. Schroeder HW, Oertel J, Gaab MR. Endoscopic treatment of cerebrospinal fluid pathway obstructions. Neurosurgery. 2008;62:1084–92. https://doi.org/10.1227/01.neu.0000333774.81563.d8.
12. Schroeder HW, Gaab MR. Endoscopic aqueductoplasty: technique and results. Neurosurgery. 1999;45:508–15.
13. Schroeder HW, Gaab MR. Intracranial endoscopy. Neurosurg Focus. 1999;6:e1.
14. Schroeder HW, Niendorf WR, Gaab MR. Complications of endoscopic third ventriculostomy. J Neurosurg. 2002;96:1032–40. https://doi.org/10.3171/jns.2002.96.6.1032.
15. Mortazavi MM, Adeeb N, Griessenauer CJ, Sheikh H, Shahidi S, Tubbs RI, et al. The ventricular system of the brain: a comprehensive review of its history, anatomy, histology, embryology, and surgical considerations. Childs Nerv Syst. 2014;30:19–35. https://doi.org/10.1007/s00381-013-2321-3.
16. Dezena RA. Atlas of endoscopic neurosurgery of the third ventricle. Basic principles for ventricular approaches and essential intraoperative anatomy. Cham: Springer International Publishing AG; 2017. https://doi.org/10.1007/978-3-319-50068-3.
17. Caemaert J, Abdullah J, Calliauw L. A multipurpose cerebral endoscope and reflections on technique and instrumentation in endoscopic neurosurgery. Acta Neurochir Suppl Wien. 1994;61:49–53.
18. Schroeder HW. A new multipurpose ventriculoscope. Neurosurgery. 2008;62:489–91. https://doi.org/10.1227/01.neu.0000316017.43668.6c.
19. Oi S, Samii A, Samii M. Frameless free-hand maneuvering of a small-diameter rigid-rod neuroendoscope with a working channel used during high-resolution imaging. Technical note. J Neurosurg Pediatr. 2005;102:113–8. https://doi.org/10.3171/ped.2005.102.1.0113.
20. Oi S. Frameless free-hand neuroendoscopic surgery – development of the finest rigid-rod neuroendoscope model to cope with the current limitations of neuroendoscopic surgery. J Neuroendoscopy. 2010;1(1)
21. Dezena RA. General principles of endoscopic neurosurgery. In: Atlas of endoscopic neurosurgery of the third ventricle. Cham: Springer; 2017. p. 35–65.

Chapter 5
General Principles of Endoscopic Third Ventriculostomy (ETV)

5.1 General Aspects

The endoscopic third ventriculostomy (ETV) is indicated mainly in obstructive hydrocephalus, being the treatment of choice for this disease in major neurosurgical centers worldwide. Its success is measured by the clinical improvement of the patient and no need for a shunt [1]. The consideration of age and etiology is decisive in the indication and success of the procedure [2]. In the long term, success factors are still uncertain, such as poor restoration of the thickness of the cortical mantle and the increase in the cephalic perimeter. It is a procedure that is currently being widely studied, especially in terms of repeating ETV in recurrences, in communicating hydrocephalus, and in complex hydrocephalus and its association with the coagulation of choroid plexus. The definition of success in ETV is the freedom of a shunt, which in itself is a new disease. The evolution and success of ETV as a procedure highlight how important technological evolution is to the development of neurosurgery [3]. Regarding age, patients over 6 months with obstructive hydrocephalus due to stenosis of the aqueduct or tumor of the posterior fossa, and without infection or previous hemorrhage, is the ideal candidate profile. In patients with communicating hydrocephalus, the result is controversial [4]. Radiologically, the ideal candidate for ETV is the presence of obstruction at some point of the ventricular system. Magnetic resonance imaging (MRI) on T2-weighted sequences with a floor of the third ventricle deviated downward is a finding of favorable outcome. A study of 403 patients [5] observed that cistern scars more than doubled the risk of failure of ETV, and an open aqueduct increased the risk of failure by 50%. The success rate is also directly proportional to the surgeon's experience and the volume of cases approached [6]. There are clinical and radiological criteria for the definition

Electronic supplementary material The online version of this chapter (https://doi.org/10.1007/978-3-030-28657-6_5) contains supplementary material, which is available to authorized users.

of success of ETV. Clinicians include the resolution of preoperative signs of elevated intracranial pressure: improvement in the level of consciousness, resolution of eye movement abnormalities, resolution of headaches, stabilization or reduction of head circumference, and reduction of fontanelle tension in infants. The radiological criteria for adequate temporal follow-up, on the other hand, include reduction or stabilization of ventricular size over a period of 3 months. The most significant change is observed in cases of acute hydrocephalus and in the reduction of the size of the third ventricle [7]. A 15% reduction in the size of the third ventricle within 1 month is considered a reliable indicator of favorable results [8]. Generally, the degree of reduction of ventricular size in the postoperative period is inversely proportional to the duration and magnitude of symptoms in the preoperative period. So, with long-standing symptoms, the postoperative ventricular reduction will be lower [9]. It was noted that sometimes the ventricular size may not show a notable reduction in postoperative imaging compared to preoperative. On the other hand, the reduction in ventricular size after may or may not indicate a successful procedure, because it will depend on the clinical profile of the patient. A greater reduction in mean ventricular size (16% vs. 7%) was observed in successful ETV results compared to failures in this procedure [10]. Special magnetic resonance imaging sequences such as phase contrast, T2-weighted studies, and more recently, 3D-space sequences are being used to evaluate the patency of the stoma [11]. Sometimes a computed tomography (CT) contrast can be utilized if there is ventricular access to an Ommaya reservoir or a similar device. Here radiopaque contrast is injected into the ventricles through the reservoir, and computed tomography is performed that will reveal the migration of the dye from the lateral ventricle to the cisterns in the case of a patent stoma. Thus, the clinical correlation is more important than the radiological correlation to determine the successful outcome. Imaging provides a reliable means to positively predict patients of course, but its use as a single entity is inadequate [12].

5.2 ETV Success Score

The Endoscopic Third Ventriculostomy Success Score (ETVSS) (Table 5.1) is the most widely used tool in predicting the successful chances of ETV [13]. For the creation of this score, it employed logistic regression techniques based on age, etiology for hydrocephalus, and previous shunting history of the patient to predict ETV success. A range from 0 (very low chance of success) to 90 (very high chance of success) is obtained for the resulting ETVSS. Progressively higher scores are given to age ranges from >1 month, 1 month to 6 months, 6 months to a year, 1 year to 10 years, and > 10 years. Post infection, intraventricular hemorrhage, myelomeningocele, and non-tectal tumors constitute the etiology. Stenosis of aqueduct and tectal tumors obtains sequentially better scores. The third arm of the scoring system comprises of previous shunt surgery and primary procedure. The addition of the shunt score, age score, and etiology score makes up the final ETVSS. Outcomes at

Table 5.1 ETV Success Score. The calculation is age + etiology + previous shunt. Chance (%) of having a successful ETV without failure at 6 months postprocedure: high ETVSS ($\geq$ 80), moderate ETVSS (50–70), and low ETVSS ($\leq$ 40)

Score	Age	Etiology	Previous shunt
0	<1mo	Postinfectious	Previous shunt
10	1mo to <6mo		No previous shunt
20		Myelomeningocele, IVH	
		Nontectal brain tumor	
30	6mo to <1 yr	Aqueductal stenosis	
		Tectal tumor, other	
40	1 yr to <10 yrs		
50	>=10 yrs		

IVH intraventricular hemorrhage

6 months of follow-up are included in this study. The results of a follow-up study across all ETVSS groups [14] indicated that as postsurgical time progresses, there is a reduction in ETV risk failure in comparison to shunt failure. Studies published for more than 20 years were reviewed by the same group of authors in 2011, and they inferred that the actual ETV success rate can be closely predicted by ETVSS [15].

5.3   Role of Patient's Age and Etiology of Hydrocephalus

ETV success rate in 21 patients of >2 years of age was examined by Baldauf et al. [16]. It was also discovered in this study that ETV success rate in children >2 years of age and suffering from obstructive hydrocephalus depends on age and etiology with an overall success rate of 43%. In 37.5% of cases, ETV was successful in newborns. After analyzing ETV carried out for 41 hydrocephalus patients >2 years of age, Sufianov et al. [17] noticed that ETV was successful in 71.4% of children between 1 and 2 years and in 75.0% of children >1 year. They concluded that ETV success in this group of patients (<2 years) depends on the third ventricular floor thickness and the age at which hydrocephalus presented. He et al. [18] have reported 16 ETV procedures that were successfully done out of 17 attempted cases of infantile hydrocephalus of varied etiology. Also, in a retrospective study by Jernigan et al. [19], a 64% failure rate was observed after ETV, and this was higher than the 40% failure seen post shunting of 5416 newborns with hydrocephalus who underwent CSF diversion either in the form of shunting or ETV. This rate was even more noticeable if ETV was done within 3 months of birth. Ogiwara et al. [20] retrospectively analyzed 23 patients >6 months of age who were treated with ETV. They suggested that in children >3 months of age, ETV can be considered as the main treatment for hydrocephalus. The International Infant Hydrocephalus Study Group has helped to improve our understanding through their preliminary results publications [21]. The comparison between ETV and shunt success in patients >2 years of age has helped in the analysis of 158 patients, and the results indicate that shunting has a better rate of success as compared to ETV (66% vs. 88% at age of 6 months). There appears to be a higher chance of success in ETV than what is found in the ETVSS, especially in patients >3 months of age. Etiology may also play an important role based on age parameters. Koch and Wagner [22] observed poorer ETV results in obstructive hydrocephalus cases apart from aqueduct stenosis as well as in the very young age group of patients. Several studies have been described for ETV in cases of post-meningitis hydrocephalus that is associated with tuberculosis which is prevalent in Africa and South Asia. A success rate between 60% and 85% of ETV has been reported in most series published [23]. ETV helps in the diversion of CSF to previously inaccessible areas and removes exudates from areas with impaired absorption, thereby helping to enhance the delivery of drug [24]. In 2009, Chugh et al. [25] suggested that ETV can be considered as the primary interventional modality in patients with tuberculous meningitis hydrocephalus especially those with long-standing disease. ETV in spina bifida patients >6 months of age after shunt failure has been shown to have a good long-term success (approximately 80%) [26]. ETV in Dandy-Walker malformation can be an effective means to achieve a reduction in hydrocephalus and is a recommended line of treatment [27]. Hydrocephalus in Chiari 1 malformation has a complex etiology which is a matter of great debate. Nevertheless, ETV usage in Chiari 1 malformation is becoming prevalent because it causes reduced obstruction of the physiological pathways of CSF flow and absorption [28]. There is a relatively higher rate of failure of ETV for craniosynostosis. Di Rocco et al. [29] treated 11 patients having craniosynostosis with hydrocephalus, and 7 of them were successful in the outcome, while the remaining 4 required shunting. A closer supervision is proposed in these scenarios. In a study of 104 pediatric patients who underwent posterior fossa surgery, 30 were developing hydrocephalus, and a success rate of >90% was found for ETV and has been suggested as the ideal treatment for hydrocephalus in such cases [30]. Apart from being the primary line of intervention for pineal region tumors, ETV has the advantage of relieving hydrocephalus as well as providing a window for biopsy and analysis of CSF and inspecting tumor seedlings and dissemination if any [31]. Also, ETV has been reported to have similar if not better results to shunting in cases of normal pressure hydrocephalus and can be recommended as a primary line of treatment [32].

5.4   ETV and Choroid Plexus Coagulation

Faivre, in 1854, and Luschka, in 1855, were the first researchers to suggest that the choroid plexus is the source of CSF [33, 34]. Cushing supported this hypothesis through intraoperative observations [35]. Extrachoroidal fluid production was suggested by Weed, in 1914, from animal studies [34]. Dandy, in 1918, demonstrated, in an animal study, that unilateral hydrocephalus was produced when the fourth ventricle was blocked, together with the access through the foramen of Monro to the contralateral plexectomized lateral ventricle [36, 37]. Furthermore, in the same year, he also demonstrated, in an animal study, that CSF was produced by the choroid plexus. Judging from this result, he carried out choroid plexus extirpation in four newborns with communicating hydrocephalus by open surgery. In this series, one infant with moderate hydrocephalus and myelomeningocele was well at 10 months of follow-up, and the other three infants, with severe hydrocephalus, died within 4 weeks after the operation [36, 37]. Later, in 1932, Dandy also used a rigid Kelly cystoscope to inspect the lateral ventricles in two hydrocephalic children [37, 38]. CPC was attempted in one case, as described in detail in 1938 [37, 39]. The technique of CPC was first described by Putnam in 1934 [37, 40]. In subsequent years, besides CPC, other surgical treatments of hydrocephalus were introduced, including ETV and extrathecal CSF shunts. In a review, there were 95 cases of CPC from 1934 to 1957. The mean mortality rate was 15%, while the mean success rate was 60%, with an average follow-up period of 8 years. On the other hand, there were 1087 cases of various kinds of CSF shunts, including 230 ventriculoperitoneal shunts (VPSs). The mean mortality rate was 10%, and the mean initial success rate was 60%, with an average follow-up time of 2 years [37]. The results of these reviews showed a shift from CPC to CSF shunts, perhaps due to poor and limited technology. However, the late complication rate for CSF shunts was 57% [37, 41]. Scarff, in 1970, published the first large series of CPC cases, his own series of 39 children treated during a 23-year period, had a 67% success rate [42]. In 1974, a series of 12 patients who underwent choroid plexectomy was reported by Milhorat. Of the 11 survivors, 8 (72%) failed and required a further shunt [43]. After this report, and a report that CPC in rhesus monkeys reduced CSF production by only 40%, the use of CPC declined in favor of the use of CSF shunts [37]. In the neuro-endoscopic literature from the 1980s to 2004, the success rate of CPC was between 30% and 52% [44–46]. In small series, two out of three cases were successful [37, 47]. Griffith, in 1986, gave a detailed account of endoscopic intracranial neurosurgery, through a report of the results of 71 patients treated by CPC with or without CSF shunt, from 1972 to 1982 [48]. The selection criteria were infants with hydrocephalus who had progressively enlarging head circumference with grossly dilated ventricles and absent superficial CSF space on CT scans. Changes that are associated with behavior were also considered. Thirty percent of the patients in this series were not shunt-dependent. The success rates were 54%, 58%, and 22% for groups with myelomeningocele and those with communicating and obstructive hydrocephalus, respectively. The same author, in 1990, further reported the results of 32 childhood hydrocephalus cases treated by CPC between 1985 and 1988 with CT scan examinations. Eighteen patients were under the age of 6 months. Patient selection was the same as that in his previous report. In addition, all patients showed marked ventricular dilatation on a preoperative CT scan [45]. In contrast to his previous series, in this series, Griffith added postoperative perfusion of the ventricular system with artificial CSF to clear the postcoagulation blood and protein released into the CSF. The average follow-up time ranged from 1 to 4 years. Fifty-two percent of the patients were shunt-independent. All those who required VPS, except for one patient, showed requirement within an interval of ≤12 weeks. Among the successful group, most of the patients showed a head circumference similar to the preoperative size [37]. Pople and Ettles, in 1995, reviewed the results of CPC in 116 children with hydrocephalus operated from 1973 to 1993 [46]. The mean age was 2 years, and the overall hydrocephalus control rate was 49.5%. A slow to moderate rate of an increase in head circumference was observed in the children with communicating hydrocephalus, and the long-term control rate was 64%. On the other hand, in the patients who presented with tense fontanelles and rapidly progressing hydrocephalus, only 35% achieved long-term control without CSF shunts, and the authors suggested that the main indication for CPC in infants was mildly progressive communicating hydrocephalus. In these patients, it seemed that the balance between the production and absorption of CSF could be restored by only a small reduction in outflow from the choroid plexus of the lateral ventricle. In contrast, CPC was not recommended for rapidly progressive hydrocephalus with acutely raised intracranial pressure [37, 46, 49]. These first experiences were quite controversial, perhaps because of technological limitations [50–52]. In the late 1990s to early 2000s, due to the advances in neurosurgical technology, the mortality rate in isolated CPC has decreased, but the key issue for its decline in clinical practice is its relative lack of efficacy [37]. The Uganda series, reported by Dr. Benjamin Warf, investigated the beneficial effect of ETV associated with CPC for the first time, again arousing interest in this technique. It was concluded that the ETV/CPC procedure was superior to ETV alone in infants younger than 1 year of age, particularly among those with non-postinfectious hydrocephalus and myelomeningocele, but longer follow-up with neurocognitive assessment was necessary [53]. Warf published his first results from ETV/CPC for children in Africa in 2005 [53]. The long-term outcome and neurocognitive outcome were reported in 2008 [54] and 2009 [55], respectively. These reports highlighted the fact that shunt dependency in children with hydrocephalus is more dangerous in developing countries than in developed countries because of the limitations in accessing competent centers in the event of shunt malfunction or infection [53]. Warf and Campbell, in 2008 [54], reported the long-term result of ETV/CPC for East African infants with hydrocephalus related to myelomeningocele. Out of 338 newborns who had myelomeningocele that was repaired before 6 months of age, 258 of them (66%) required treatment for hydrocephalus after a follow-up of >6 months. There were 93 patients (mean age, 3 months) who had completed ETV/CPC with >1 month of follow-up. A success (shunt-independent) rate of 76% was achieved. This success rate was higher in ETV/CPC patients than in those with ETV alone for infants aged 6 months or younger with hydrocephalus in association with myelomeningocele, as reported in the literature [26, 56]. Warf et al. [55], in 2009, reported the ventricular volume and neurocognitive outcome in children with myelomeningocele and who have been treated for hydrocephalus in Uganda. The modified Bayley Scales of Infant Development (BSID-III) and the frontal/occipital horn ratio (FOR) were used to compare three groups of patients with myelomeningocele. For the modified BSID-III, there was a statistically significant difference between the treatment groups with VPS and those with ETV/CPC. For the ventricular size, the FOR was 0.7, 0.65, and 0.62 for the VPS, ETV/CPC, and the treatment-not required group, respectively, without a statistically significant difference between the groups. The authors suggested that future research is needed to compare outcomes by using a larger control group of children treated primarily with VPS [55]. Even so, Warf et al. have applied ETV/CPC to encephalocele, with a success rate of 85% [57], and in obstructive hydrocephalus due to aqueductal stenosis, they have achieved a success rate of 81.9% in patients treated by ETV/CPC [58]. Dandy-Walker complex is another condition that is treatable by ETV/CPC, according to Warf's African series [59]. Treating this disease by neuroendoscopy in the Uganda scenario was reported on a wide range. Therefore, using this method instead of the traditional standard of creating shunt dependence as the primary management is of great importance. This disease has a success rate of 73%, 74%, and 100% for Dandy-Walker variant, Dandy-Walker malformation, and mega cisterna magna, respectively. Eighty-eight percent of the patients were younger than 12 months, and 95% had an open aqueduct at the time of the ETV/CPC. None required posterior fossa shunting in a mean follow-up of 24.2 months [60]. From the same Warf's African series, the use of ETV/CPC in communicating hydrocephalus was a viable option [60]. ETV/CPC was significantly more successful than ETV alone in treating congenital idiopathic hydrocephalus of infancy. In this study with 64 infants (mean/median age, 6.1/5.0 months), 16 consecutive patients were treated by ETV alone and the subsequent 48 by ETV/CPC (mean/median follow-up 34.4/36.0 months). ETV was successful in 20% and ETV/CPC in 72.4% at 4 years ($p < 0.0002$, log-rank test; $p = 0.0006$, Gehan-Breslow-Wilcoxon test; hazard ratio 6.9, 95% confidence interval [CI] 2.5–19.3). It was assumed that the primary effect of ETV, as a pulsation absorber, and of CPC, as a pulsation reducer, may be to reduce the net force of the intraventricular pulsations that produce ventricular expansion. On the other hand, ETV alone may be less successful for infants because of their greater brain compliance. Nevertheless, this technique appears to have a higher long-term success rate and a lower infection rate than primary shunt placement and should be considered an effective primary treatment option for congenital idiopathic hydrocephalus [60]. A new predictor of ETV/CPC success arose from the Uganda series: the CCHU (CURE Children's Hospital of Uganda) ETV Success Score. With this model, clinicians can correctly identify children that have a good chance of successful outcome with ETV, considering the special features and conditions of the Ugandan population [61] (Table 5.2).

An early North American multicenter experience with ETV/CPC in infants demonstrates that the procedure has reasonable safety in selected cases. The degree of CPC achieved might be associated with a surgeon's learning curve, and this appears

Table 5.2 CCHU ETV Success Score. The calculation is age + etiology + choroid plexus coagulation. Chance (%) of having success: 7–9 (high chance of success), 3–6 (moderate chance of success), 0–2 (low chance of success)

Score	Age	Etiology	Choroid plexus cauterization
0	<6mo	Other	None
1	6mo to <1 yr	Postinfectious	
2		Myelomeningocele	Partial unilateral
3	1 yr or older		
4			Complete bilateral

to affect success, suggesting that surgeon training might improve results [62]. Of note, both the ETV Success Score and the CCHU ETV Success Score predicted success following ETV/CPC in a single-center North American cohort of patients [63]. For complex or multiloculated hydrocephalus, choroid plexus coagulation or its resection in conjunction with multiple septal fenestration and CSF shunt is a good option to control hydrocephalus. In a review of their series of 93 cases of multiloculated hydrocephalus, Zuccaro and Ramos [64] reported that choroid plexus coagulation and its resection were performed in 14 cases (8 by endoscopy and 6 by craniotomy). In another review, Zhu and Di Rocco concluded that, because of the variable success rate, each patient must be studied individually [37]. Initial experience with ETV/CPC for post-hemorrhagic hydrocephalus of prematurity has revealed the importance of the prepontine cistern status and the predictive value of fast imaging employing steady-state acquisition (FIESTA) MRI [65]. ETV/CPC as an initial procedure is safe and eliminates the need for a CSF shunt in premature infants with hydrocephalus and intraventricular hemorrhage (IVH). Although, with a low success rate of 37%, compared with shunt treatment, there is a reduced rate of complications occurring which may justify this procedure in the initial management of hydrocephalus. Because some of the factors studied have been shown to have influence on the outcome, the selection of patient based on these observations might help to increase the success rate [66]. Besides the combined ETV/CPC technique, nowadays there are new indications for isolated CPC, such as in extreme hydrocephalus and hydranencephaly [47, 67, 68]. As a result of the fragility and thinness of the scalp, avoiding a CSF shunt is advisable in these conditions as well as the common presence of infected scalp ulcers at the parietal bosses. In 2004, Morota and Fujiyama described a unilateral transmural approach technique for bilateral CPC, in which they used a flexible neuroendoscope for three infants with IVH related to hydrocephalus. Two of the patients were shunt-independent. The authors suggested that the characteristics of favorable candidates for CPC were severely advanced hydrocephalus, such as hydranencephalic hydrocephalus, slow progressive hydrocephalus, and lack of/or thinned-out septum pellucidum to make the bilateral endoscopic access possible [47]. Malheiros et al., in 2010, in a series of 17 patients, carried out CPC in 9 patients; the procedure successfully controlled excessive head circumference and signs of increased intracranial pressure in 8 of these patients (88.8%). One endoscopic procedure in a hydranencephalic child failed after 7 months, resulting in VPS placement. There were no complications related to this method of treatment. The authors concluded that CPC is an acceptable alternative to VPS for the treatment of hydranencephaly and near hydranencephaly, because it is a single, definitive, safe, effective, and economical treatment that may avoid the complications of shunting [67]. In another recent study, in severe congenital hydrocephalus and hydranencephaly, CPC stabilized macrocephaly in approximately 40% of the infants who had the procedure and was considered as an alternative to VPS placement. A follow-up of 30–608 days (median, 120 days) was done for patients. Out of the 30 patients that were evaluated, 13 (43.3%) had successful CPC, including 5 of 10 patients with hydranencephaly and 8 of 20 with severe hydrocephalus. In

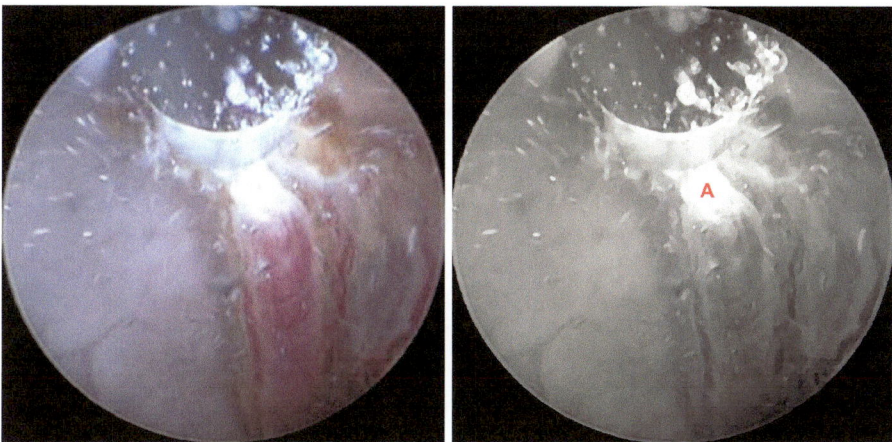

Fig. 5.1 (A) Bipolar coagulation of the lateral posterior choroidal artery. (Reprinted from Dezena [69]. With permission from Springer Nature)

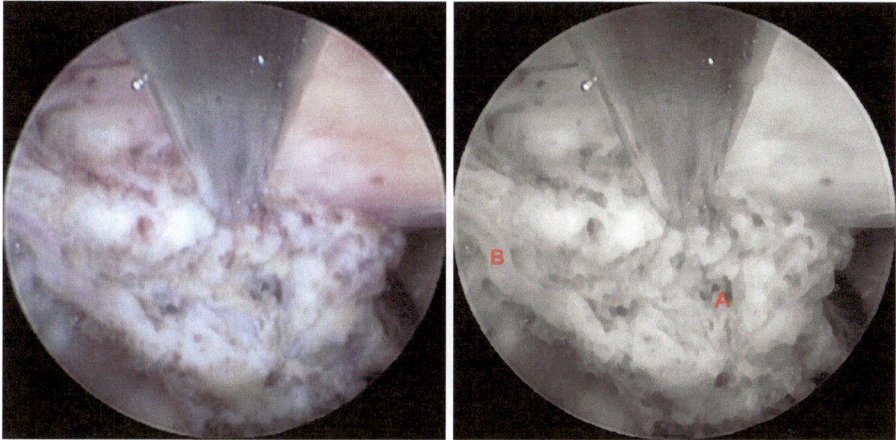

Fig. 5.2 (A) Coagulation of the choroid glomus, (B) coagulated lateral posterior, choroidal artery. (Reprinted from Dezena [69]. With permission from Springer Nature)

14 (82%) of the 17 failed patients, CPC failure resulting from increased head circumference was evident and from CSF leakage in 3. There were 13 failures that occurred within 3 months of surgery out of 17. Six patients died: 3 and 2 whose CPC procedures were failures and successful, respectively, and 1 postoperatively. Ten patients out of 17 in whom CPC failed underwent VPS insertion. We can conclude from this African study that CPC stabilizes macrocephaly when isolated and can be considered as an alternative to CSF shunt placement [68]. Figures 5.1 and 5.2 and online video 5.1 demonstrate choroid plexus coagulation.

References

1. Deopujari CE, Karmarkar VS, Shaikh ST. Endoscopic third ventriculostomy: success and failure. J Korean Neurosurg Soc. 2017;60(3):306–14. https://doi.org/10.3340/jkns.2017.0202.013.
2. Dezena RA. Atlas of endoscopic neurosurgery of the third ventricle. Basic principles for ventricular approaches and essential intraoperative anatomy. Cham: Springer International Publishing AG; 2017. https://doi.org/10.1007/978-3-319-50068-3.
3. Schmitt PJ, Jane JA Jr. A lesson in history: the evolution of endoscopic third ventriculostomy. Neurosurg Focus. 2012;33:E11.
4. Rangel-Castilla L, Barber S, Zhang YJ. The role of endoscopic third ventriculostomy in the treatment of communicating hydrocephalus. World Neurosurg. 2012;77:555–60.
5. Warf BC, Kulkarni AV. Intraoperative assessment of cerebral aqueduct patency and cisternal scarring: impact on success of endoscopic third ventriculostomy in 403 African children. J Neurosurg Pediatr. 2010;5:204–9.
6. Egger D, Balmer B, Altermatt S, Meuli M. Third ventriculostomy in a single pediatric surgical unit. Childs Nerv Syst. 2010;26:93–9.
7. Santamarta D, Martin-Vallejo J, Díaz-Alvarez A, Maillo A. Changes in ventricular size after endoscopic third ventriculostomy. Acta Neurochir (Wien). 2008;150:119–27; discussion 127.
8. Schwartz TH, Yoon SS, Cutruzzola FW, Goodman RR. Third ventriculostomy: post-operative ventricular size and outcome. Minim Invasive Neurosurg. 1996;39:122–9.
9. Schwartz TH, Ho B, Prestigiacomo CJ, Bruce JN, Feldstein NA, Goodman RR. Ventricular volume following third ventriculostomy. J Neurosurg. 1999;91:20–5.
10. Kulkarni AV, Drake JM, Armstrong DC, Dirks PB. Imaging correlates of successful endoscopic third ventriculostomy. J Neurosurg. 2000;92:915–9.
11. Algin O, Ucar M, Ozmen E, Borcek AO, Ozisik P, Ocakoglu G, et al. Assessment of third ventriculostomy patency with the 3D-SPACE technique: a preliminary multicenter research study. J Neurosurg. 2015;122:1347–55.
12. Buxton N, Turner B, Ramli N, Vloeberghs M. Changes in third ventricular size with neuroendoscopic third ventriculostomy: a blinded study. J Neurol Neurosurg Psychiatry. 2002;72:385–7.
13. Kulkarni AV, Drake JM, Mallucci CL, Sgouros S, Roth J, Constantini S, Canadian Pediatric Neurosurgery Study Group. Endoscopic third ventriculostomy in the treatment of childhood hydrocephalus. J Pediatr. 2009;155:254–259.e1.
14. Kulkarni AV, Drake JM, Kestle JR, Mallucci CL, Sgouros S, Constantini S. Canadian Pediatric Neurosurgery Study Group: predicting who will benefit from endoscopic third ventriculostomy compared with shunt insertion in childhood hydrocephalus using the ETV success score. J Neurosurg Pediatr. 2010;6:310–5.
15. Kulkarni AV, Riva-Cambrin J, Browd SR. Use of the ETV success score to explain the variation in reported endoscopic third ventriculostomy success rates among published case series of childhood hydrocephalus. J Neurosurg Pediatr. 2011;7:143–6.
16. Baldauf J, Oertel J, Gaab MR, Schroeder HW. Endoscopic third ventriculostomy in children younger than 2 years of age. Childs Nerv Syst. 2007;23:623–6.
17. Sufianov AA, Sufianova GZ, Iakimov IA. Endoscopic third ventriculostomy in patients younger than 2 years: outcome analysis of 41 hydrocephalus cases. J Neurosurg Pediatr. 2010;5:392–401.
18. He Z, An C, Zhang X, He X, Li Q. The efficacy analysis of endoscopic third ventriculostomy in infantile hydrocephalus. J Korean Neurosurg Soc. 2015;57:119–22.
19. Jernigan SC, Berry JG, Graham DA, Goumnerova L. The comparative effectiveness of ventricular shunt placement versus endoscopic third ventriculostomy for initial treatment of hydrocephalus in infants. J Neurosurg Pediatr. 2014;13:295–300.
20. Ogiwara H, Dipatri AJ Jr, Alden TD, Bowman RM, Tomita T. Endoscopic third ventriculostomy for obstructive hydrocephalus in children younger than 6 months of age. Childs Nerv Syst. 2010;26:343–7.

21. Kulkarni AV, Sgouros S, Constantini S, IIHS Investigators. International infant hydrocephalus study: initial results of a prospective, multicenter comparison of endoscopic third ventriculostomy (ETV) and shunt for infant hydrocephalus. Childs Nerv Syst. 2016;32:1039–48.
22. Koch D, Wagner W. Endoscopic third ventriculostomy in infants of less than 1 year of age: which factors influence the outcome? Childs Nerv Syst. 2004;20:405–11.
23. Figaji AA, Fieggen AG, Peter JC. Endoscopic third ventriculostomy in tuberculous meningitis. Childs Nerv Syst. 2003;19:217–25.
24. Jonathan A, Rajshekhar V. Endoscopic third ventriculostomy for chronic hydrocephalus after tuberculous meningitis. Surg Neurol. 2005;63:32–4; discussion 34–35.
25. Chugh A, Husain M, Gupta RK, Ojha BK, Chandra A, Rastogi M. Surgical outcome of tuberculous meningitis hydrocephalus treated by endoscopic third ventriculostomy: prognostic factors and postoperative neuroimaging for functional assessment of ventriculostomy. J Neurosurg Pediatr. 2009;3:371–7.
26. Teo C, Jones R. Management of hydrocephalus by endoscopic third ventriculostomy in patients with myelomeningocele. Pediatr Neurosurg. 1996;25:57–63; discussion 63.
27. Hu CF, Fan HC, Chang CF, Wang CC, Chen SJ. Successful treatment of Dandy-Walker syndrome by endoscopic third ventriculostomy in a 6-month-old girl with progressive hydrocephalus: a case report and literature review. Pediatr Neonatol. 2011;52:42–5.
28. Di Rocco C, Frassanito P, Massimi L, Peraio S. Hydrocephalus and Chiari type I malformation. Childs Nerv Syst. 2011;27:1653–64.
29. Di Rocco F, Jucá CE, Arnaud E, Renier D, Sainte-Rose C. The role of endoscopic third ventriculostomy in the treatment of hydrocephalus associated with faciocraniosynostosis. J Neurosurg Pediatr. 2010;6:17–22.
30. Tamburrini G, Pettorini BL, Massimi L, Caldarelli M, Di Rocco C. Endoscopic third ventriculostomy: the best option in the treatment of persistent hydrocephalus after posterior cranial fossa tumour removal? Childs Nerv Syst. 2008;24:1405–12.
31. Morgenstern PF, Souweidane MM. Pineal region tumors: simultaneous endoscopic third ventriculostomy and tumor biopsy. World Neurosurg. 2013;79(2 Suppl):S18.e9–e13.
32. Gangemi M, Maiuri F, Buonamassa S, Colella G, de Divitiis E. Endoscopic third ventriculostomy in idiopathic normal pressure hydrocephalus. Neurosurgery. 2004;55:129–34; discussion 134.
33. Cserr HF. Physiology of the choroid plexus. Physiol Rev. 1971;51:273–311.
34. Weed LH. Studies on cerebro-spinal fluid. No. IV: the dual source of cerebro-spinal fluid. J Med Res. 1914;31:93–118.
35. Cushing H. Studies on the cerebrospinal fluid. I Introduction. J Med Res. 1914;31:1–19.
36. Dandy WE. Extirpation of the choroids plexus of the lateral ventricles in communicating hydrocephalus. Ann Surg. 1918;68:569–79.
37. Zhu X, Di Rocco C. Choroid plexus coagulation for hydrocephalus not due to CSF overproduction: a review. Childs Nerv Syst. 2013;29:35–42. https://doi.org/10.1007/s00381-012-1960-0.
38. Dandy WE. The brain. Hagerstown: W. F. Prior Company; 1932.
39. Dandy WE. The operative treatment of communicating hydrocephalus. Ann Surg. 1938;108:194–202.
40. Putnam TJ. Treatment of hydrocephalus by endoscopic coagulation of choroid plexuses: description of a new instrument and preliminary report of results. N Engl J Med. 1934;210:1373–6.
41. Scarff JE. Evaluation of treatment of hydrocephalus. Results of third ventriculostomy and endoscopic cauterization of choroid plexuses compared with mechanical shunts. Arch Neurol. 1966;14:382–91.
42. Scarff JE. The treatment of nonobstructive (communicating) hydrocephalus by endoscopic cauterization of the choroid plexuses. J Neurosurg. 1970;33:1–18.
43. Milhorat TH. Failure of choroid plexectomy as treatment for hydrocephalus. Surg Gynecol Obstet. 1974;139:505–8.
44. Griffith HB. Endoneurosurgery: endoscopic intracranial surgery. Proc R Soc Lond B. 1977;195:261–8.

45. Griffith HB, Jamjoom AB. The treatment of childhood hydrocephalus by choroid plexus coagulation and artificial cerebrospinal fluid perfusion. Br J Neurosurg. 1990;4:95–100.
46. Pople IK, Ettles D. The role of endoscopic choroid plexus coagulation in the management of hydrocephalus. Neurosurgery. 1995;36:698–701.
47. Morota N, Fujiyama Y. Endoscopic coagulation of choroid plexus as treatment for hydrocephalus: indication and surgical technique. Childs Nerv Syst. 2004;20:816–20. https://doi.org/10.1007/s00381-004-0936-0.
48. Griffith HB. Endoneurosurgery: endoscopic intracranial surgery. Adv Tech Stand Neurosurg. 1986;14:2–24.
49. Philips MF, Shanno G, Duhaime AC. Treatment of villous hypertrophy of the choroid plexus by endoscopic contact coagulation. Pediatr Neurosurg. 1998;28:252–6.
50. Dezena RA, Pereira CU, Araújo LP, Ribeiro MP, Oliveira HA. Neuroendoscopic choroid plexus coagulation for pediatric hydrocephalus: review of historical aspects and rebirth. J Bras Neurocirurg. 2014;25:30–5.
51. Dezena RA. The rebirth of neuroendoscopic choroid plexus coagulation as treatment of pediatric hydrocephalus. J Neurol Stroke. 2014;1:00012.
52. Dezena RA. Neuroendoscopic choroid plexus coagulation in the current pediatric neurosurgery. J Neurosurg Sci. 2016;60:287–8.
53. Warf BC. Comparison of endoscopic third ventriculostomy alone and combined with choroid plexus cauterization in infants younger than 1 year of age: a prospective study in 550 African children. J Neurosurg. 2005;103:475–81. https://doi.org/10.3171/ped.2005.103.6.0475.
54. Warf BC, Campbell JW. Combined endoscopic third ventriculostomy and choroid plexus cauterization as primary treatment of hydrocephalus for infants with myelomeningocele: long-term results of a prospective intent-to-treat study in 115 East African infants. J Neurosurg Pediatr. 2008;2:310–6. https://doi.org/10.3171/PED.2008.2.11.310.
55. Warf B, Ondoma S, Kulkarni A, Donnelly R, Ampeire M, Akona J, et al. Neurocognitive outcome and ventricular volume in children with myelomeningocele treated for hydrocephalus in Uganda. J Neurosurg Pediatr. 2009;4:564–70. https://doi.org/10.3171/2009.7.PEDS09136.
56. Kadrian D, van Gelder J, Florida D, Jones R, Vonau M, Teo C, et al. Long-term reliability of endoscopic third ventriculostomy. Neurosurgery. 2005;56:1271–8.
57. Warf BC, Stagno V, Mugamba J. Encephalocele in Uganda: ethnic distinctions in lesion location, endoscopic management of hydrocephalus, and survival in 110 consecutive children. J Neurosurg Pediatr. 2011;7:88–93. https://doi.org/10.3171/2010.9.PEDS10326.
58. Warf BC, Tracy S, Mugamba J. Long-term outcome for endoscopic third ventriculostomy alone or in combination with choroid plexus cauterization for congenital aqueductal stenosis in African infants. J Neurosurg Pediatr. 2012;10:108–11. https://doi.org/10.3171/2012.4.PEDS1253.
59. Warf BC, Dewan M, Mugamba J. Management of Dandy-Walker complex associated infant hydrocephalus by combined endoscopic third ventriculostomy and choroid plexus cauterization. J Neurosurg Pediatr. 2011;8:377–83. https://doi.org/10.3171/2011.7.PEDS1198.
60. Warf BC. Congenital idiopathic hydrocephalus of infancy: the results of treatment by endoscopic third ventriculostomy with or without choroid plexus cauterization and suggestions for how it works. Childs Nerv Syst. 2013;29:935–40. https://doi.org/10.1007/s00381-013-2072-1.
61. Warf BC, Mugamba J, Kulkarni AV. Endoscopic third ventriculostomy in the treatment of childhood hydrocephalus in Uganda: report of a scoring system that predicts success. J Neurosurg Pediatr. 2010;5:143–8. https://doi.org/10.3171/2009.9.PEDS09196.
62. Kulkarni AV, Riva-Cambrin J, Browd SR, Drake JM, Holubkov R, Kestle JR, et al. Endoscopic third ventriculostomy and choroid plexus cauterization in infants with hydrocephalus: a retrospective Hydrocephalus Clinical Research Network study. J Neurosurg Pediatr. 2014;14:224–9. https://doi.org/10.3171/2014.6.
63. Weil AG, Fallah A, Chamiraju P, Ragheb J, Bhatia S. Endoscopic third ventriculostomy and choroid plexus cauterization with a rigid neuroendoscope in infants with hydrocephalus. J Neurosurg Pediatr. 2015;30:1–11. https://doi.org/10.3171/2015.5.PEDS14692.

64. Zuccaro G, Ramos JG. Multiloculated hydrocephalus. Childs Nerv Syst. 2011;27:1609–19. https://doi.org/10.1007/s00381-011-1528-4.
65. Warf BC, Campbell JW, Riddle E. Initial experience with combined endoscopic third ventriculostomy and choroid plexus cauterization for post-hemorrhagic hydrocephalus of prematurity: the importance of prepontine cistern status and the predictive value of FIESTA MRI imaging. Childs Nerv Syst. 2011;7:1063–71.
66. Chamiraju P, Bhatia S, Sandberg DI, Ragheb J. Endoscopic third ventriculostomy and choroid plexus cauterization in posthemorrhagic hydrocephalus of prematurity. J Neurosurg Pediatr. 2014;13:433–9. https://doi.org/10.3171/2013.12.PEDS13219.
67. Malheiros JA, Trivelato FP, Oliveira MM, Gusmão S, Cochrane DD, Steinbok P. Endoscopic choroid plexus cauterization versus ventriculoperitoneal shunt for hydranencephaly and near hydranencephaly:a prospective study. Neurosurgery. 2010;66:459–64. https://doi.org/10.1227/01.NEU.0000365264.99133.CA.
68. Shitsama S, Wittayanakorn N, Okechi H, Albright AL. Choroid plexus coagulation in infants with extreme hydrocephalus or hydranencephaly. J Neurosurg Pediatr. 2014;14:55–7. https://doi.org/10.3171/2014.3.PEDS13488.
69. Dezena RA. Entering the third ventricle: the lateral ventricle. In: Atlas of endoscopic neurosurgery of the third ventricle. Cham: Springer; 2017. p. 69–119.

Chapter 6
Surgical Technique of Endoscopic Third Ventriculostomy (ETV)

6.1 Opening Tuber Cinereum

The ventricular access point to the ETV is Kocher's point, which is located approximately 2 cm lateral to the midline and 2 cm anterior to the coronal suture [1]. After the endoscope enters the lateral ventricle, the foramen of Monro is visualized, which is the main point of orientation for all ventricular endoscopic procedures. Through this portal the third ventricle is reached, and the anterior segment, particularly the mammillary bodies, should be located next. The exact site for fenestration is preferably at the midpoint between the mammillary bodies and the infundibular recess. Obviously this position can vary according to the position of the structures below the tuber cinereum, especially the basilar artery [1]. For fenestration, bipolar coagulation can be used through heat or even opening with the coagulator deactivated through mechanical compression. Grasping forceps or Fogarty balloon catheter can also be used. There is no consensus on the best way to perform fenestration. It is believed that the use of monopolar energy can induce an inflammatory response, which can contribute to the closure of the ostomy. Laser may be a good option [2]. The appropriate size of the stoma is usually around 3–4 mm in diameter. An approximate estimate of size adequacy is the ability to insert the endoscope into the interpeduncular cistern. The diameter of the stoma is increased with a Fogarty balloon catheter of 2, 3, or 4 Fr. This is an important step during the procedure. An additional advantage is mechanical compression over small capillary bleeds that may occur during fenestration (Figs. 6.1 and 6.2). Of extreme importance for the success of the ETV, besides the opening of the tuber cinereum, is the opening of the membrane of Liliequist, which is an arachnoid layer that is located below the third ventricle and delimits the interpeduncular and prepontine cisterns [1, 3]. Standard ETV is showed in Videos 6.1, 6.2, 6.3, 6.4, 6.5, 6.6, 6.7, 6.8, 6.9, 6.10, 6.11, and 6.12.

Electronic supplementary material The online version of this chapter (https://doi.org/10.1007/978-3-030-28657-6_6) contains supplementary material, which is available to authorized users.

© Springer Nature Switzerland AG 2020
R. A. Dezena, *Endoscopic Third Ventriculostomy*,
https://doi.org/10.1007/978-3-030-28657-6_6

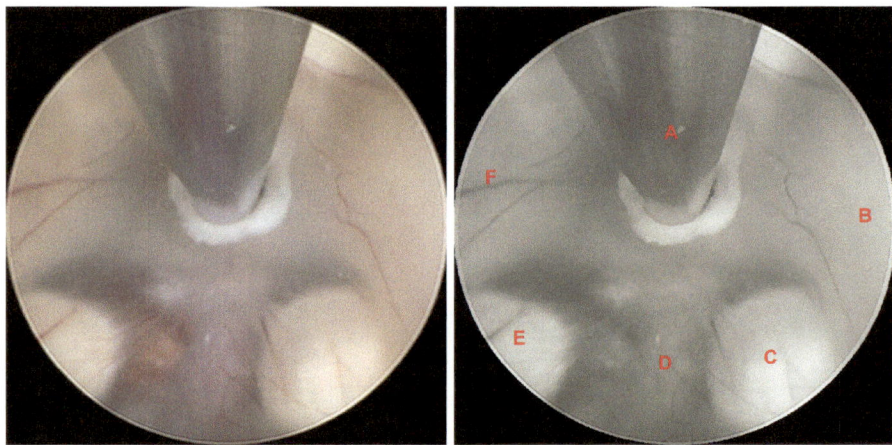

Fig. 6.1 Opening tuber cinereum. (A) Bipolar coagulation electrode, (B) right hypothalamus, (C) right mammillary body, (D) basilar artery under premammillary recess, (E) left mammillary body, (F) left hypothalamus. (Reprinted from Dezena [30]. With permission from Springer Nature)

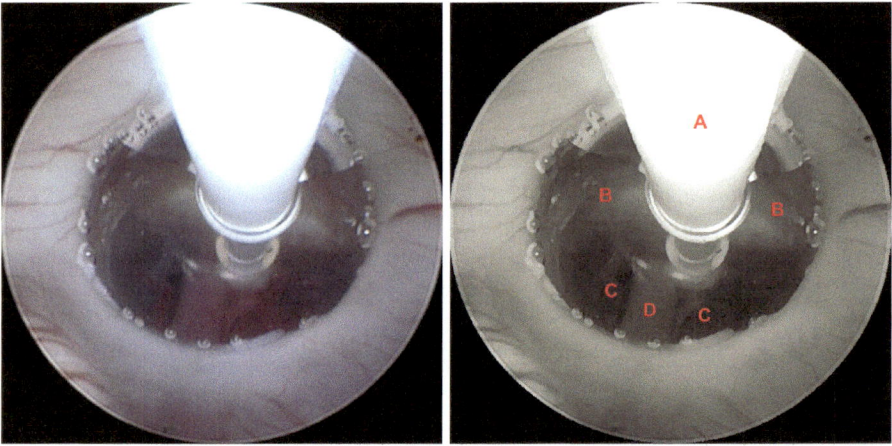

Fig. 6.2 Ostomy dilatation. (A) Fogarty balloon catheter dilatation, (B) dorsum sellae, (C) pontine branches of the basilar artery, (D) basilar artery. (Reprinted from Dezena [30]. With permission from Springer Nature)

6.2   Membrane of Liliequist (ML)

The ML is a small structure of arachnoid tissue located in the basal cisterns of the brain, inferiorly to the third ventricle and anteriorly to the brainstem. This structure separates the interpeduncular cistern from the chiasm, superiorly, and from the prepontine cistern, inferiorly. The ML is located precisely in a position just below the floor of the third ventricle, being an arachnoid slide, without vascularization. The

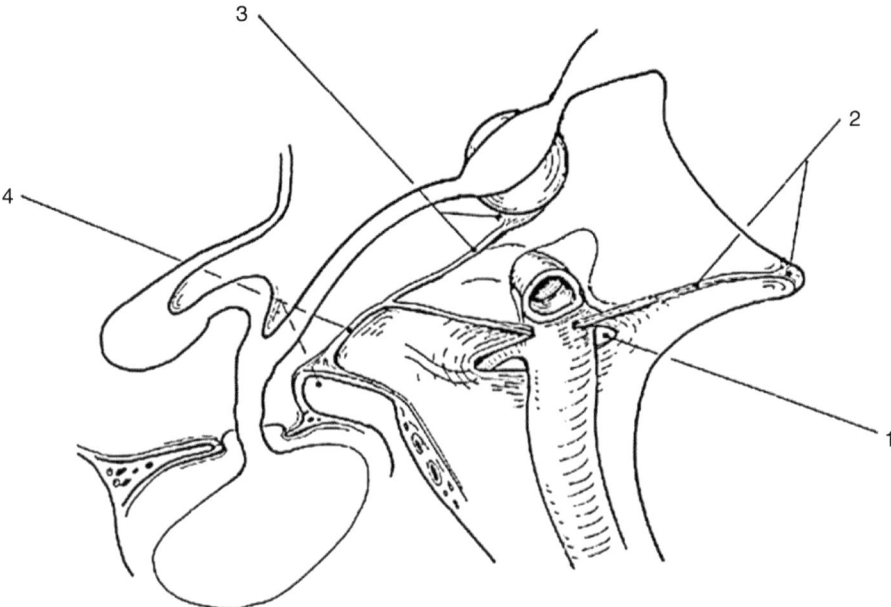

Fig. 6.3 Membrane of Liliequist. Gap of mesencephalic portion (1), mesencephalic portion (2), diencephalic portion (3), common part and its insertion at dorsum sellae (4). (Reprinted from Seeger and Zentner [31]. With permission from Springer Nature)

membrane is divided into two portions: the upper one (diencephalic), which is inserted anteriorly to the mammillary bodies, and the inferior one (mesencephalic), which extends to the mesencephalic-pons groove [1]. The diencephalic portion anteriorly separates the chiasmatic cistern from the interpeduncular cistern. Posteriorly this same portion divides the interpeduncular cistern into an upper segment (*pars profunda*) and a lower segment (*pars superficialis*) (Figs. 6.3, 6.4, and 6.5). The mesencephalic portion establishes the boundaries between the interpeduncular and prepontine cisterns, being thinner, incomplete, or fenestrated and being perforated by the basilar artery. The diencephalic portion, on the other hand, forms a continuous structure, and its opening during the ETV is extremely necessary [1, 3] (Fig. 6.6). Rhoton, in a commentary on the diencephalic portion, describes it as firmer and without perforations, which acts as a barrier to the passage of air or other substances through the subarachnoid space, besides describing that such portion is fixed to the posterior margin of the mammillary bodies [1, 3]. After performing ETV, the interpeduncular and prepontine cisterns should be inspected to discard any arachnoid membrane that may interfere in the circulation of the cerebrospinal fluid. The ineffective opening of the ML may lead to failure of the LVT, that is, the flow of CSF coming from the third ventricle may be blocked [3–5]. The lateral margins of the ML are fixed to the arachnoid around the oculomotor nerve or directly on it, but the membrane may extend beyond the oculomotor nerve [1, 3]. On the other

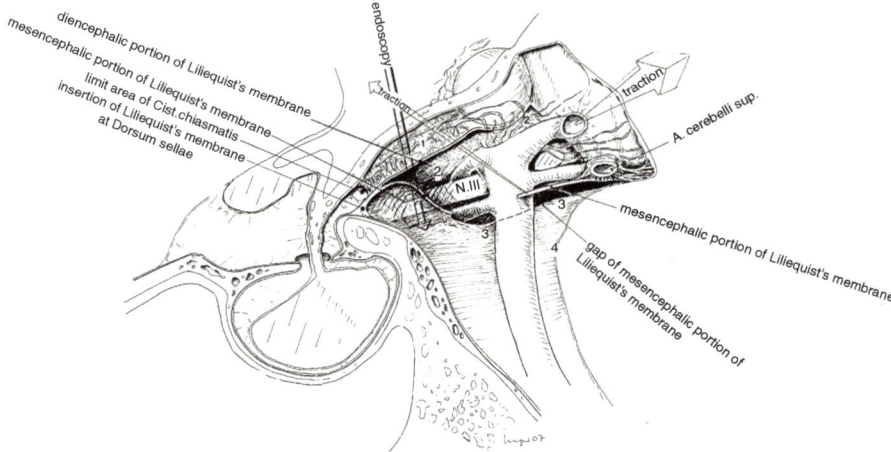

Fig. 6.4 Detail of the membrane of Liliequist just below the third ventricle. *Pars profunda* of the interpeduncular cistern (1), *pars superficialis* of the interpeduncular cistern (2), prepontine cistern (3), and pia mater (4). (Reprinted from Seeger [32]. With permission from Springer Nature)

Fig. 6.5 Sagittal T2-weighted magnetic resonance imaging (MRI) depicting the membrane of Liliequist and cisterns below the third ventricle. Ependymal layer (A), pars profunda of the interpeduncular cistern (B), diencephalic portion of the membrane of Liliequist (C), pars superficialis of the interpeduncular cistern (D), mesencephalic portion of the membrane of Liliequist (E), prepontine cistern (F), insertion of the membrane of Liliequist at the dorsum sellae (G). (Reprinted from Dezena [33]. With permission from Springer Nature)

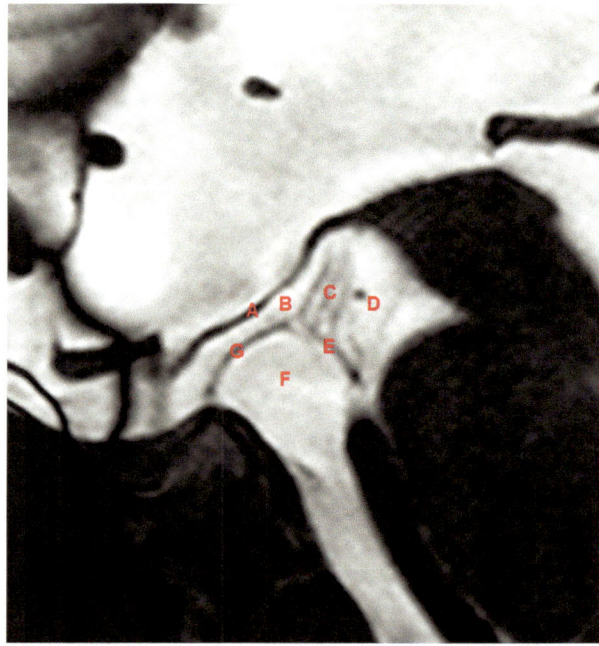

hand, it has been described that the ML may be located between the back posterior clinoid process and the retromammillary space. This finding has implications on the success of the ETV, since in a retromammillary fixation, it is less important to fenestrate the ML, because there would already be a communication between the third ventricle and interpeduncular cistern, and only the fenestration of the floor of the

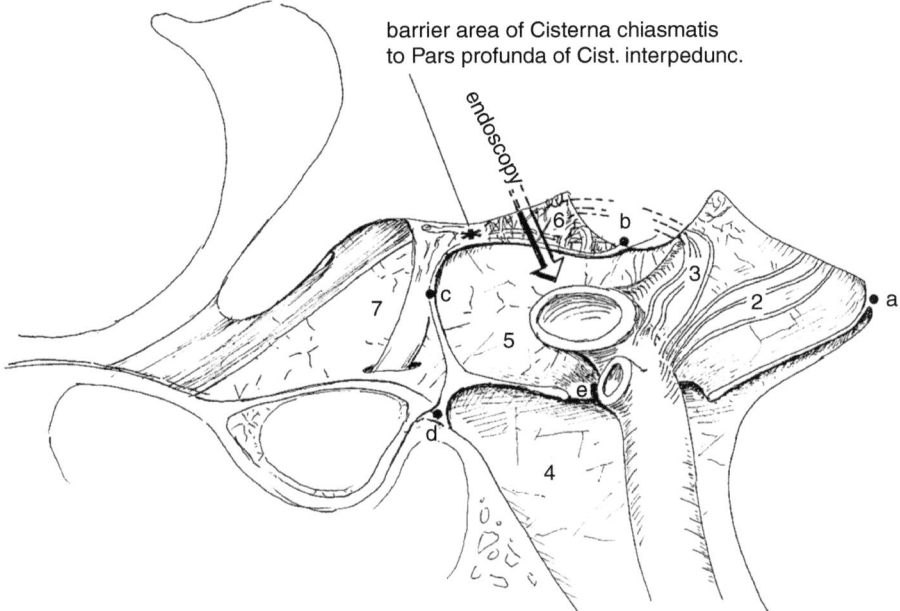

Fig. 6.6 Trajectory of the neuroendoscope through the pars profunda of the interpeduncular cistern. This step is mandatory for ETV success. Insertion of the mesencephalic portion of the membrane of Liliequist at the pontomesencephalic rim (a), insertion of the diencephalic portion of the membrane of Liliequist at mammillary body (b), bulging of this segment against the chiasmatic cistern (c), insertion of the membrane of Liliequist at the dorsum sellae (d), gap of the mesencephalic segment (e). Bifurcation of the basilar artery (1), posterior bundle of the thalamoperforating arteries, penetrating the posterior perforated substance (2), anterior bundle of the thalamoperforating arteries, crossing pars superficialis of the interpeduncular cistern (3), prepontine cistern (4), pars superficialis of the interpeduncular cistern (5), pars profunda of the interpeduncular cistern (6), chiasmatic cistern (7). (Reprinted from Seeger [32]. With permission from Springer Nature)

third ventricle is necessary [1, 6, 7]. The initial description of the subarachnoid space was performed by the anatomists Blasius, Ruysch, and Vieussens, in the seventeenth century, who considered all arachnoid membranes as a single structure, similar to a large continuous envelope that covered the brain [8]. This space was also studied by Bichat in 1800, who demonstrated that it is a structure with complex anatomy and trabeculation and also found to be not only a single membrane, as previously described. Also worthy of note are the work of Magendie, from 1842, who described the communication between the ventricular system and the subarachnoid space, and the classic description of Key and Retzius who studied the arachnoid system with dyes injected into the ventricles [9]. The works of Bengt Liliequist are from 1956 to 1959 that, from pneumoencephalography in human cadavers, described unequivocally the ML, which received its name [8]. Since the 1970s their interest has been accentuated by the advancement of microneurosurgery, which began to use the cisternal space as a natural and atraumatic pathway for various brain structures. Yasargil, in 1976, described the anatomy of subarachnoid cisterns from the observation of 1500 microsurgical procedures, citing the term "membrane of Liliequist" and consecrating the eponym [10]. The first endoscopic views are from the early 2000s. Vinas and Panigrahi (2001) injected 20 brains with silicone and performed microscopic dissection of the ML, enumerating several controversies of anatomical descriptions previously performed, besides being the pioneers in describing the endoscopic view of the membrane [11]. Lu and Zhu (2005) described the anatomy of the interpeduncular cistern from the microscopic dissection of eight human cadavers and showed the relationship of the membranes with the bifurcation of the basilar artery, the oculomotor nerves, the posterior cerebral arteries, the perforating arteries, and other structures [12]. Sufianov et al. (2009) dissected the ML microscopically and examined pieces of brain sections to study the interpeduncular cistern. They described the membrane in detail, adding to the description the diencephalic and mesencephalic portions [13]. Qi et al. (2011) restudied the membranes of the interpeduncular cistern from the dissection of 20 human cadavers, emphasizing the presence of the mesencephalic portion in its anterior portion [14]. Wang et al. (2011) studied the three-dimensional structure of the membrane in order to assist in the anatomical understanding by the minimally invasive technique. They described again the diencephalic and mesencephalic portions and added a pair of hypothalamic portions. However, they emphasized that all would only be present in two thirds of the specimens [15]. After the development of the neuroendoscopic technique and the popularization of the ETV, the attention of researchers focused on the anatomical characteristics of the membrane under this aspect. Buxton et al. (1998) described the case of a child with a Chiari II malformation, submitted to a failed ETV. It was necessary to follow the procedure and open a membrane below the floor of the third ventricle. They emphasized the relationship of the anatomy classically described of the portions of LM, the need to recognize them and open them in ETV [16]. Froelich et al. (2008) tried to understand the relationship between neuroendoscopic vision and anatomy. They studied 13 heads, initially with endoscopic exploration and later by microscopy. Their conclusions were that the membrane may present as a single membrane in most cases, or two parts, the diencephalic and mesencephalic portions [17]. Inoue et al. (2009) studied the anatomy of cisterns trying to maintain their integrity, through micro and endoscopic study of 22 brains of human cadavers. They described this anatomy by identifying 9 cisterns and 20 internal arachnoid membranes, including ML. These authors cited their two portions, emphasizing the relationship with the other structures and their appearance on the endoscopic perspective. They also produced images that showed their vision through a neuroendoscope [18]. Anik et al. (2011) studied 24 fresh adult human cadavers, exploring the membrane by microscopy and, subsequently, the cisterns with rigid endoscope. They stated that in 18 specimens, the membrane was divided into two classical portions. They also described its relationship with neighboring structures [19]. Zhang et al. (2012) dissected 24 heads of human cadavers formolized with microscopic technique and histological study. They reported the ML as consisting of two portions, always having lateral extension adhered to the edge of the tentorium. Half of the specimens were adhered to the medial portion of the hippocampal uncus. They also clarified that the oculomotor nerve would be below the most superior portion of the membrane, adhered to it by a membrane of its own. They also showed endoscopic transoperative photographs exemplifying the findings [20]. Dezena (2015) described the ML from transoperative observations, showing photographic images of the two main portions and their relationship with the structures present in the cisterns [21]. Fushimi et al. (2003) described three portions of LM from the 3D magnetic resonance imaging (MRI) study of 31 healthy volunteers. The authors identified the membrane in all patients and showed anatomical variations. On MRI interpretation, the thickness of the membrane was less than half the thickness of the floor of the third ventricle in 88% of the volunteers [22]. Anik et al. (2011) studied flow MRI in 51 children under 2 years of age, submitted to ETV, verifying whether this examination could predict the method efficacy index. They concluded that the presence of flow in the interpeduncular cisterns and prepontine are predictive factors of success [23]. Anik et al. (2011) studied 29 conventional MRI of adult patients submitted to ETV and restudied with the 3D technique after the operation. The membrane was identified in all cases. Of the 21% in which the ETV failed, they observed that the non-open membrane was responsible for three of these failures [24]. Etus et al. (2011) studied the structure of the membrane by biopsy in 11 patients with hydrocephalus, 5 of recent onset and 6 of long duration. They concluded that in chronic cases, there is degeneration of the membrane with the appearance of collagen and fibroblasts, which would make it dense and difficult to be opened. The same finding was not found in acute cases. They inferred that when degeneration occurs, there may be a greater possibility of failure due to incorrect opening of the membrane [25]. Yadav et al. (2012) described the technique of ETV with emphasis on the importance of opening the ML and stated that failures in the procedure may occur because it is not considered during surgery [26]. Romero et al. (2014) analyzed the videos of ETV of 51 patients (27 adults and 24 children). They established a score based on transoperative findings: anatomical distortion, surgical accidents, open ML with two maneuvers, multiple subarachnoid membranes, absence or weak pulsation of the floor and flexible premammillary membrane that required coagulation. They established the statistical possibility of factors that could determine failure and concluded that the association of these factors increases the possibility of failure. Individually in each patient, the need for maneuver to open the Liliequist membrane was a relevant factor for failure [27]. Mortazavi et al. (2014) reviewed the anatomical description. And they concluded that its real anatomical nature is still the subject of debate. However, they demonstrated that in a variable portion of times, it may be absent (15–42.9%). They also compiled findings from other authors regarding the diencephalic portion stating that, in most cases, it would be thick and transparent. These authors also correlated the findings with the ETV, drawing attention to situations in which its opening may not be important (retromamillary position). However, they emphasized that the ML or any arachnoid structure below third ventricle must be opened to successfully

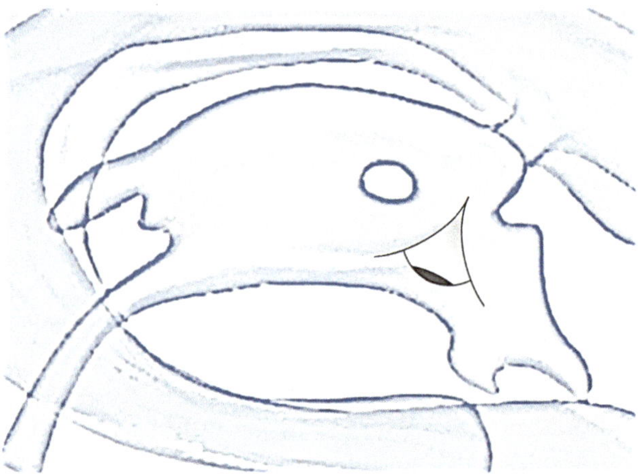

Fig. 6.7 Direction of the endoscopic viewing angle for interpeduncular and prepontine cisterns

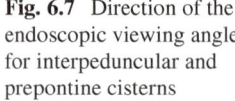

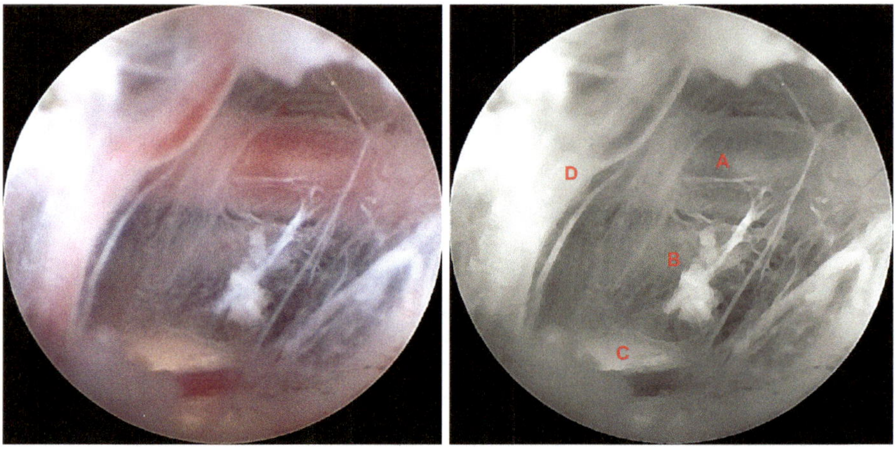

Fig. 6.8 (A) Right posterior cerebral artery (P1), (B) membrane of Liliequist, (C) pons under membrane of Liliequist, (D) thalamoperforating artery. (Reprinted from Dezena [30]. With permission from Springer Nature)

complete the surgery. They also considered the possibility of jointly opening the floor and the ML, without identifying it, especially in long-term hydrocephalus, stating that, in most cases, only the opening of the diencephalic portion would be sufficient for success. However, they affirmed that, sometimes, the interpeduncular cistern is a closed space, and it is ideal to also open the mesencephalic portion [28]. Schulte-Altedorneburg et al. (2016) retrospectively studied the MRI of 37 adult patients with hydrocephalus, trying to identify all portions of the ML, concluding that the membrane is visible half the time [29]. Next, images of the ML are shown from the best endoscopic viewing angle of the interpeduncular and prepontine cisterns (Fig. 6.7) and intraoperative images of diencephalic and mesencephalic and portions (Figs. 6.8, 6.9, and 6.10).

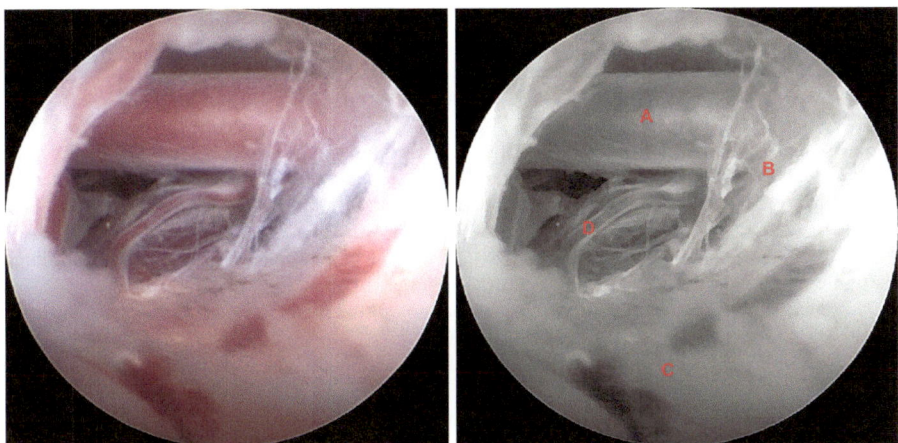

Fig. 6.9 (A) Right posterior cerebral artery (P1), (B) membrane of Liliequist, (C) tuber cinereum, (D) thalamoperforating artery. (Reprinted from Dezena [30]. With permission from Springer Nature)

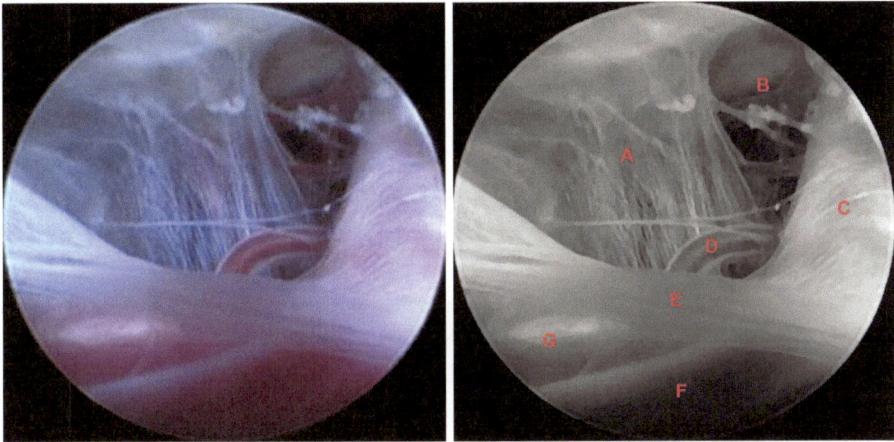

Fig. 6.10 (A) Membrane of Liliequist, mesencephalic portion; (B) prepontine cistern; (C) basilar artery, (D) pontine arterial branch; (E) membrane of Liliequist, diencephalic portion; (F) left posterior cerebral artery (P1); (G) left superior cerebellar artery. (Reprinted from Dezena [33]. With permission from Springer Nature)

References

1. Dezena RA. Atlas of endoscopic neurosurgery of the third ventricle. In: Basic principles for ventricular approaches and essential intraoperative anatomy. 1th ed. Cham: Springer International Publishing AG; 2017. https://doi.org/10.1007/978-3-319-50068-3-1.
2. Devaux BC, Joly LM, Page P, Nataf F, Turak B, Beuvon F, et al. Laser-assisted endoscopic third ventriculostomy for obstructive hydrocephalus: technique and results in a series of 40 consecutive cases. Lasers Surg Med. 2004;34(5):368–78.

3. Deopujari CE, Karmarkar VS, Shaikh ST. Endoscopic third ventriculostomy: success and failure. J Korean Neurosurg Soc. 2017;60(3):306–14. https://doi.org/10.3340/jkns.2017.0202.013.
4. Vogel TW, Bahuleyan B, Robinson S, Cohen AR. The role of endoscopic third ventriculostomy in the treatment of hydrocephalus. J Neurosurg Pediatr. 2013;12(1):54–61. https://doi.org/10.3171/2013.4.PEDS12481.
5. Tubbs RS, Hattab EM, Loukas M, Chern JJ, Wellons M, Wellons JC III, et al. Histological analysis of the third ventricle floor in hydrocephalic and nonhydrocephalic brains: application to neuroendocrine complications following third ventriculostomy procedures. J Neurosurg Pediatr. 2012;9(2):178–81. https://doi.org/10.3171/2011.11.PEDS11290.
6. Seeger W, Zentner J. Anatomical basis of cranial neurosurgery. 1th ed. Cham: Springer International Publishing AG; 2018. https://doi.org/10.1007/978-3-319-63597-2.
7. Seeger W. Endoscopic and microsurgical anatomy of the upper basal cisterns. Wien: Springer; 2008. https://doi.org/10.1007/978-3-211-77035-1.
8. Connor DE Jr, Nanda A. Bengt Liliequist: life and accomplishments of a true renaissance man. J Neurosurg. 2016;126(2):1–5.
9. Key A, Retzius MG. Studien in der Anatomie des Nervensystems und des Bindegewebes. Stockholm: Samson and Wallin; 1875.
10. Yasargil MG, Kasdaglis K, Jain KK, Weber HP. Anatomical observations of the subarachnoid cisterns of the brain during surgery. J Neurosurg. 1976;44(3):298–302.
11. Vinas FC, Panigrahi M. Microsurgical anatomy of the Liliequist's membrane and surrounding neurovascular territories. Minim Invasive Neurosurg. 2001;44(2):104–9.
12. Lü J, Zhu X. Microsurgical anatomy of the interpeduncular cistern and related arachnoid membranes. J Neurosurg. 2005;103(2):337–41.
13. Sufianov AA, Sufianova GZ, Iakimov IA. Microsurgical study of the interpeduncular cistern and its communication with adjoining cisterns. Childs Nerv Syst. 2009;25(3):301–8. https://doi.org/10.1007/s00381-008-0746-x.
14. Qi ST, Fan J, Zhang XA, Pan J. Reinvestigation of the ambient cistern and its related arachnoid membranes: an anatomical study. J Neurosurg. 2011;115(1):171–8. https://doi.org/10.3171/2011.2.JNS101365.
15. Wang SS, Zheng HP, Zhang FH, Wang RM. Microsurgical anatomy of Liliequist's membrane demonstrating three-dimensional configuration. Acta Neurochir. 2011;153(1):191–200. https://doi.org/10.1007/s00701-010-0823-2.
16. Buxton N, Vloeberghs M, Punt J. Liliequist's membrane in minimally invasive endoscopic neurosurgery. Clin Anat. 1998;11(3):187–90.
17. Froelich SC, Abdel Aziz KM, Cohen PD, van Loveren HR, Keller JT. Microsurgical and endoscopic anatomy of Liliequist's membrane: a complex and variable structure of the basal cisterns. Neurosurgery. 2008;63(1 Suppl 1):ONS1–8; discussion ONS8-9. https://doi.org/10.1227/01.neu.0000335004.22628.
18. Inoue K, Seker A, Osawa S, Alencastro LF, Matsushima T, Rhoton AL Jr. Microsurgical and endoscopic anatomy of the supratentorial arachnoidal membranes and cisterns. Neurosurgery. 2009;65(4):644–64; discussion 665. https://doi.org/10.1227/01.NEU.0000351774.81674.32.
19. Anik I, Ceylan S, Koc K, Tugasaygi M, Sirin G, Gazioglu N, et al. Microsurgical and endoscopic anatomy of Liliequist's membrane and the prepontine membranes: cadaveric study and clinical implications. Acta Neurochir. 2011;153(8):1701–11. https://doi.org/10.1007/s00701-011-0978-5.
20. Zhang XA, Qi ST, Huang GL, Long H, Fan J, Peng JX. Anatomical and histological study of Liliequist's membrane: with emphasis on its nature and lateral attachments. Childs Nerv Syst. 2012;28(1):65–72. https://doi.org/10.1007/s00381-011-1599-2.
21. Dezena R. Endoscopic views of the membrane of Liliequist. J Bras Neurocirurg. 2015;26(4):320–3.
22. Fushimi Y, Miki Y, Ueba T, Kanagaki M, Takahashi T, Yamamoto A, et al. Liliequist membrane: three-dimensional constructive interference in steady state MR imaging. Radiology. 2003;229(2):360–5; discussion 365.

23. Anik I, Ceylan S, Koc K, Anık Y, Etus V, Genc H. Role of interpeduncular and prepontine cistern cerebrospinal fluid flow measurements in prediction of endoscopic third ventriculostomy success in pediatric triventricular hydrocephalus. Pediatr Neurosurg. 2010;46(5):344–50. https://doi.org/10.1159/000323413.

24. Anik I, Ceylan S, Koc K, Anık Y, Etus V, Genc H. Membranous structures affecting the success of endoscopic third ventriculostomy in adult aqueductus sylvii stenosis. Minim Invasive Neurosurg. 2011;54(2):68–74. https://doi.org/10.1055/s-0031-1277172.

25. Etus V, Solakoglu S, Ceylan S. Ultrastructural changes in the Liliequist membrane in the hydrocephalic process and its implications for the endoscopic third ventriculostomy procedure. Turkish Neurosurg. 2011;21(3):359–66. https://doi.org/10.5137/1019-5149.JTN.4171-11.0.

26. Yadav YR, Parihar V, Pande S, Namdev H, Agarwal M. Endoscopic third ventriculostomy. J Neurosci Rural Pract. 2012;3(2):163–73. https://doi.org/10.4103/0976-3147.98222.

27. Romero L, Ros B, Ibáñez G, Ríus F, González L, Arráez M. Endoscopic third ventriculostomy: can we predict success during surgery? Neurosurg Rev. 2014;37(1):89–97. https://doi.org/10.1007/s10143-013-0494-6.

28. Mortazavi MM, Rizq F, Harmon O, Adeeb N, Gorjian M, Hose N, et al. Anatomical variations and neurosurgical significance of Liliequist's membrane. Childs Nerv Syst. 2015;31(1):15–28. https://doi.org/10.1007/s00381-014-2590-5.

29. Schulte-Altedorneburg G, Linn J, Kunz M, Brückmann H, Zausinger S, Morhard D. Visualization of Liliequist's membrane prior to endoscopic third ventriculostomy. Radiol Med. 2016;121(3):200–5. https://doi.org/10.1007/s11547-015-0588-z.

30. Dezena RA. Inside the third ventricle. In: Atlas of endoscopic neurosurgery of the third ventricle. Cham: Springer; 2017. p. 121–208.

31. Seeger W, Zentner J. Anatomical base of surgery. In: Anatomical basis of cranial neurosurgery. Cham: Springer; 2018. p. 19–74.

32. Seeger W. Topography of basal cisterns (figs. 14 to 30). In: Endoscopic and microsurgical anatomy of the upper basal cisterns. Vienna: Springer; 2008. p. 5–8.

33. Dezena RA. Beyond the third ventricle: inside the interpeduncular and prepontine cisterns. In: Atlas of endoscopic neurosurgery of the third ventricle. Cham: Springer; 2017. p. 209–36. With permission from Springer Nature.

Chapter 7
Alternative Technique: Endoscopic Transseptumpellucidumrostrostomy (ETSPR)

7.1 Introduction

In certain situations, endoscopic third ventriculostomy (ETV) may be difficult to perform, such as in cases of thickening of the floor of the third ventricle and anatomical variations in the interpeduncular cistern by inflammatory reaction making it difficult to identify the anatomical parameters and perforation of the floor or when the interpeduncular cistern is reduced or occupied by an ectatic basilar artery. Therefore, alternatives to endoscopic fenestrations, diverting and restoring the CSF flow, are extremely useful. This chapter aims to present a study of the anatomical viability of performing a communication between the ventricular system and the longitudinal fissure of the brain, by means of fenestration of the rostral lamina of the corpus callosum, and establish the anatomical parameters for its performance as a surgical procedure by an endoscopic route. Historically, surgical techniques to treat hydrocephalus due to obstructions of the CSF circulation were described before the identification of communications between the ventricular system and other compartments. In 1922, Dandy performed the opening of the lamina terminalis by craniotomy, communicating the third ventricle with the longitudinal fissure of the brain [1–3]. Mixter, in 1923, performed the first endoscopic third ventriculostomy (ETV), fenestrating the floor of the third ventricle, communicating it with the interpeduncular cistern [2–4]. Contemporary authors used the opening of the lamina terminalis in brain aneurysm clipping surgeries and observed a reduction in the incidence of hydrocephalus due to subarachnoid hemorrhage [5–9]. In 2003, Nakao and Itakura described the opening of the lamina terminalis with a flexible endoscope to treat a hydrocephalus secondary to tubercular meningitis [10], and since then the procedure has become a viable alternative in the treatment of hydrocephalus due to ventricular obstruction. Another internal derivation pathway described through the endoscopic pathway is the communication of the third ventricle with the quadrigeminal cistern, through the suprapineal recess [11]. Therefore, the knowledge of alternative internal derivations of the ventricular system presents its value in the endoscopic treatment of hydrocephalus, especially in those cases in which the endoscopic third ventriculostomy is not a plausible alternative. Empirical observations of ventricular catheters of functional derivations accidentally positioned in the longitudinal fissure of the brain are evidence that such space can function as an internal endoscopic derivation pathway.

7.2   Methodology

7.2.1   Anatomical Landmarks of Frontal Horn and Longitudinal Fissure

In this study, 16 brain specimens obtained from autopsies were used, which had a normal appearance in the initial macroscopic inspection. Nine were female and seven were male, ages ranging from 13 to 69 years (43.5 + _13.14) and weights ranging from 940 to 1533 grams (1162.7 + _148.75). The brains were fixed in 10% formalin and sectioned in a median sagittal plane from the corpus callosum to the brainstem and cerebellum, separating the pericallosal arteries, the two leaflets of the septum pellucidum, the lateral walls of the third ventricle, and the fornix columns and, in addition, sectioning the anterior commissure, the lamina terminalis, the interthalamic adhesion, the floor of the third ventricle between the mammillary bodies, and the optic chiasm in the midline. The anterior cerebral arteries were maintained adhered to their natural bed in each hemisphere. After the sagittal section, the following anatomical structures were identified in each hemisphere (Fig. 7.1): the corpus callosum and its divisions, the interventricular foramen, the fornix column, the lamina terminalis, the supraoptic recess, the mammillary bodies, the tuber cinereum, the paraterminal gyrus, and the anterior cerebral artery. The central groove, the precentral gyrus, and the precentral groove were identified in the convexity of the hemispheres, and then a point was marked about 4 cm anterior to the precentral groove and 3 cm from the midline, which was used as a reference to perform trepanning (Fig. 7.2). To measure the distances between the anatomical structures, needles were positioned on the rostrum, genu, body, and splenium of the corpus callosum, on the supraoptic recess, and on the tuber cinereum, located anteriorly to the mammillary bodies, on the floor of the third ventricle. The portion of the rostrum of the corpus callosum that was thinner and laminar, adjacent to the lower part of the septum pellucidum, was identified as the rostral lamina [12], which has as its posterior limit the fornix column. The interventricular foramen was identified in the posterior part of the fornix column and in its posterior wall of the foramen. Two landmarks were identified and marked in the anterior cerebral arteries: the first at the origin of the anterior communicating artery and the second at the first flexure of its A2

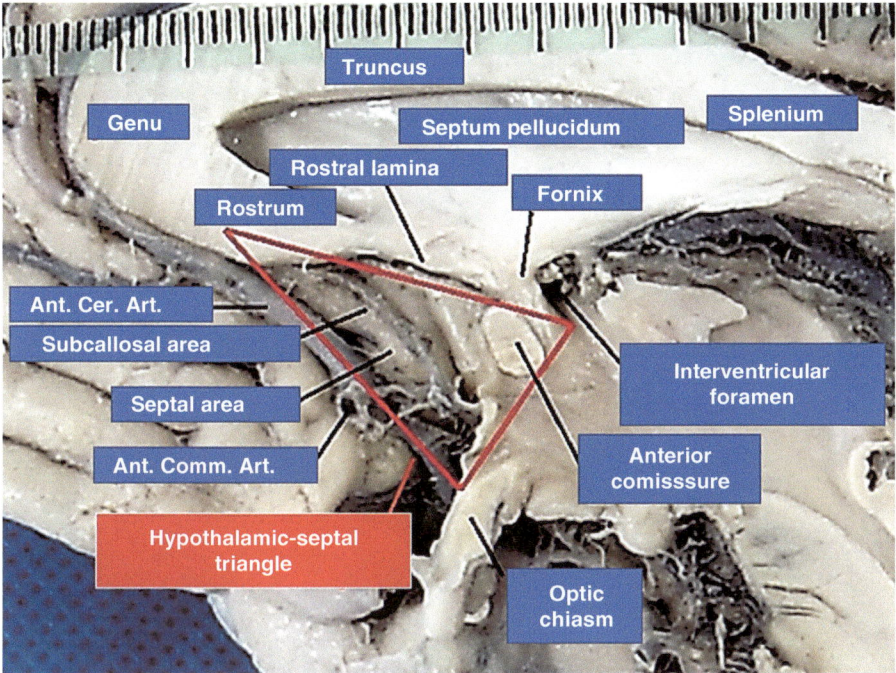

Fig. 7.1 Midline sagittal section of the brain showing the rostral lamina, hypothalamic-septal triangle, and neighbor structures. (Reprinted from Fuziki et al. [1]. With permission from Acta Cirurgica Brasileira)

portion, at the site of alteration of the ascending path to the anterior, below the rostrum of the corpus callosum. Subsequently, each cerebral hemisphere was sectioned in an axial section, parallel to the junction of the septum pellucidum with the corpus callosum. With this section, a superior view of the floor of the lateral ventricle was obtained, maintaining the medial wall of the lateral ventricle formed by each leaflet of the septum pellucidum. Needles were inserted at the following points of reference (Fig. 7.3): at the beginning of the rostral lamina, at the limit between the rostral lamina and the fornix column, and at the posterior limit of the fornix column with the interventricular foramen. According to the anatomical points marked, the following measurements were performed (Fig. 7.4): length of the rostral lamina, anterior-posterior diameter of the interventricular foramen, anterior-posterior diameter of the fornix column, height of the septum pellucidum (craniocaudal axis), thickness of the rostrum of the corpus callosum, distance from the interventricular foramen to the tuber cinereum, distance from the rostral lamina to the supraoptic recess, distance from the rostral lamina to the anterior communicating artery, and distance from the rostral lamina to the anterior cerebral artery.

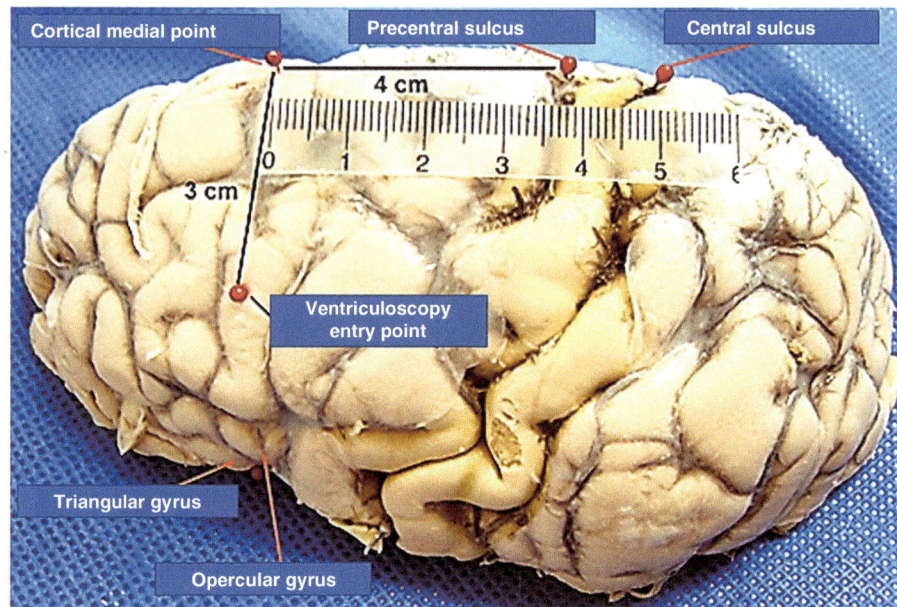

Fig. 7.2 Superior view of a left brain hemisphere. Identification of the central sulcus, precentral sulcus, cortical medial point, corticotomy's entry point to ventriculoscopy, triangular gyrus, and opercular gyrus. (Reprinted from Fuziki et al. [1]. With permission from Acta Cirurgica Brasileira)

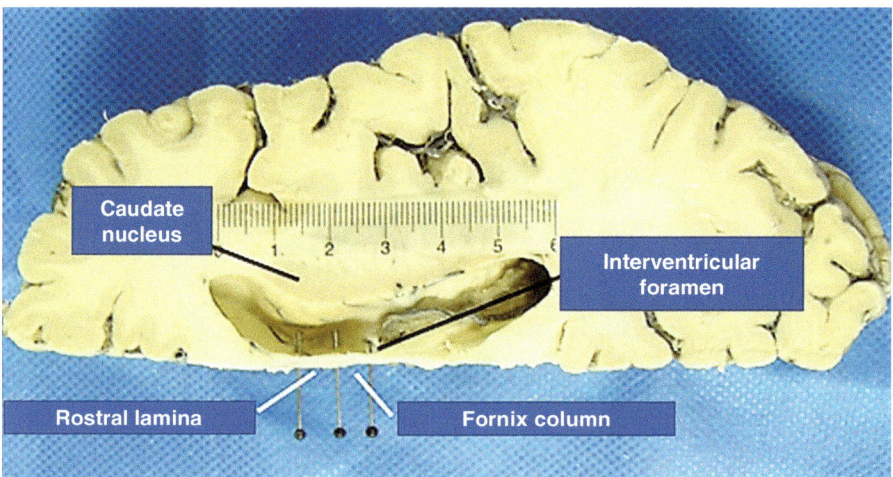

Fig. 7.3 Superior view of an axial section through the lateral ventricle with needles marking the anterior border of the interventricular foramen/fornix column and the fornix column/rostral lamina border. (Reprinted from Fuziki et al. [1]. With permission from Acta Cirurgica Brasileira)

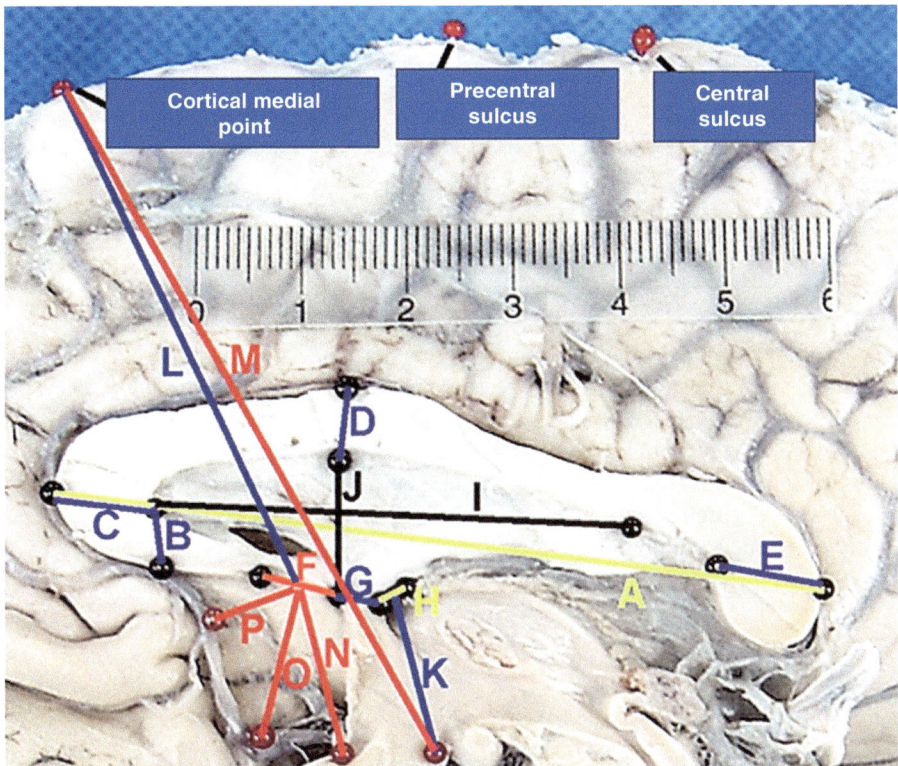

Fig. 7.4 Midline sagittal section of the brain showing the measured lines. (A) Rostrum/splenium line; (B) rostrum thickness; (C) genu thickness; (D) body thickness; (E) splenium thickness; (F) rostral lamina length; (G) fornix column thickness; (H) interventricular foramen diameter; (I) lateral ventricle length; (J) septum pellucidum height; (K) interventricular foramen to tuber cinereum distance; (L) cortex to rostral lamina distance; (M) cortex to tuber cinereum distance; (N) rostral lamina/supraoptic recess distance; (O) rostral lamina/anterior communicating artery distance; (P) rostral lamina/anterior cerebral artery distance. (Reprinted from Fuziki et al. [1]. With permission from Acta Cirurgica Brasileira)

7.2.2   Endoscopic Fenestration from Lateral Ventricle

The brains that presented slightly dilated ventricles were reconstructed using methacrylate glue, carefully, to allow visualization of the pellucid septum, the rostrum of the corpus callosum, the third ventricle, and the original positions of the anterior cerebral and anterior communicating arteries. Prior to reconstitution, in each of the hemispheres, a tunnel-shaped corticectomy was performed from a cortical point located 4 cm anterior to the precentral groove and 3 cm lateral to the midline and followed toward the interventricular foramen, to perform ventriculoscopy and ostomy in the septum pellucidum and in the rostral lamina, based on the parameters obtained. The endoscopic procedure was performed with a rigid MINOP endoscope (Aesculap AG, Tuttlingen, Germany) with a diameter of 2.7 mm, with 4 working channels, with 6 mm trocar, with a 0° lens, and with 2 mm forceps for grasping and dissection, coupled to a video recording system. After the procedure, the brains were sectioned again in the sagittal and axial planes to study the ostomy by direct visualization.

7.2.3 Statistical Analysis

The variances and means of the measurements made were compared interhemispheres, the variances with the F test and the means with the Student's t test for paired observations, accepting as significant values $p < 0.05$. Pearson's correlation tests were also performed between the interventricular diameter and the anterior-posterior diameter of the fornix column and between the anterior-posterior diameter of the interventricular foramen and the length of the rostral lamina. Statistical tests were performed using Office Excel 2003 (Microsoft, USA).

7.3 Results

7.3.1 Measurements of Anatomical Landmarks of Frontal Horn and Longitudinal Fissure

The measurements of the distances between the anatomical references located on the floor of the frontal horn of the lateral ventricle and in the hypothalamic-septal triangle are presented in Table 7.1. There was no significant difference between the measurements made in the two cerebral hemispheres ($p < 0.05$, F test for variance and

Table 7.1 Rates and standard deviations of measures performed between anatomical points close to hypothalamic-septal triangle

	Hemispheres	
	Right	Left
Rostral lamina length	7,07 ± 1,22 mm	7,12 ± 0,82 mm
Interventricular foramen diameter	4,84 ± 0,66 mm	5,03 ± 0,55 mm
Fornix column diameter	5,74 ± 0,92 mm	5,82 ± 0,98 mm
Corpus callosum rostrum thickness	6,89 ± 1,47 mm	6,7 ± 0,9 mm
Interventricular foramen/tuber cinereum distance	18,14 ± 2,86 mm	17,76 ± 2,9 mm
Rostral lamina/supraoptic recess distance	16,65 ± 2,55 mm	16,08 ± 2,84 mm
Rostral lamina/anterior communicating artery distance	15,33 ± 2,6 mm	15,95 ± 2,73 mm
Rostral lamina/anterior cerebral artery distance	8,62 ± 2,0 mm	8,76 ± 1,72 mm

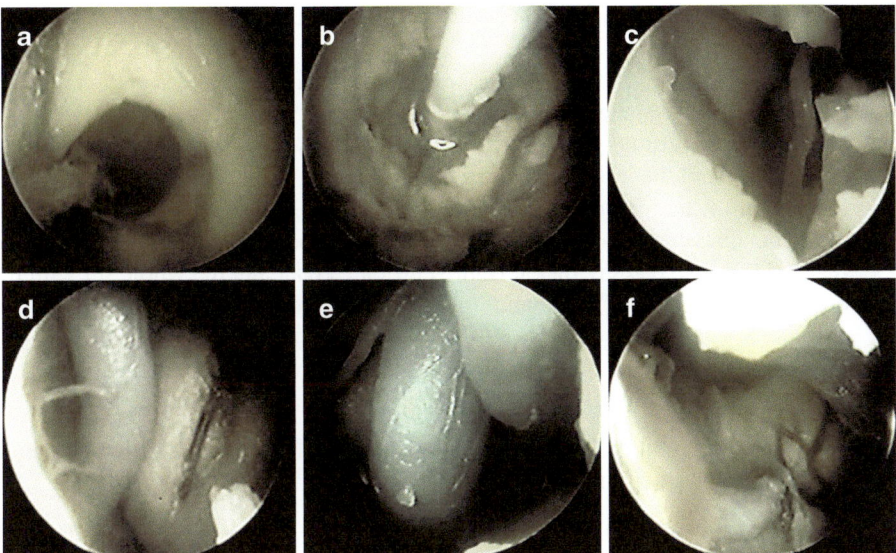

Fig. 7.5 Images of experimental endoscopic procedure. (**a**) Interventricular foramen; (**b**) fenestration enlargement by Fogarty balloon catheter; (**c**) subcallosal area; (**d**) left anterior cerebral artery; (**e**) left and right anterior cerebral arteries; (**f**) optic chiasm

Student's t test for paired observations between means). Positive correlations were observed between the anteroposterior diameter of the interventricular foramen and the anterior-posterior diameter of the fornix column (Pearson's correlation coefficient $R = 0.35$) and between the anterior-posterior diameter of the interventricular foramen and the length of the rostral lamina (Pearson's correlation coefficient $R = 0.23$). With the values of the right and left hemispheres, the mean values were calculated for the anterior-posterior diameter of the interventricular foramen (4.93 mm + _ 0.60), anterior-posterior diameter of the fornix column (5.78 mm + _ 0.93), and the length of the rostral lamina (7.09 mm + _ 1.02). Based on these parameters, the point for performing the ETSPR was defined as a point anterior the limit of the interventricular foramen with the fornix column, at a distance proportional to twice the anterior-posterior diameter of the interventricular foramen, at a crossroads with the limit between the lower portion of the septum pellucidum and the floor of the frontal horn.

7.3.2 Endoscopic Fenestration from Lateral Ventricle

The steps followed to perform the transseptumpellucidumrostrostomy with endoscopic technique were (Fig. 7.5):

- Identification of the interventricular foramen, fornix column, septum pellucidum, and septal vein in the right lateral ventricle
- Location of the point previously defined to perform the ostomy

- Perforation of the septum pellucidum and floor of the frontal horn with 2.0 mm forceps
- Enlargement of the ostomy with movements to open the forceps and then with 3F Fogarty balloon catheter
- Inspection by ostomy with identification of the left subcallosal area, the subcallosal artery, and the left anterior cerebral artery
- Inspection of the ostomy through the left lateral ventricle with visualization of the right subcallosal area and the left anterior cerebral artery
- Inspection of the ostomy by the right ventricle, advancing the whole set with the optics visualizing the right and left anterior cerebral arteries and the optic chiasm
- Final inspection of the transseptumpellucidumrostrostomy with visualization of the left and right ventricles

After performing the ETSPR in the two anatomical specimens, the examination of the ostomy presented the following characteristics:

- Previously there was a small advance of the dissection of 2–3 mm beyond the rostral lamina reaching a small portion of the rostrum of the corpus callosum (Fig. 7.6).
- Subsequently, the limit of the ostomy was approximately 5 mm in front of the fornix spine (Fig. 7.6).
- Laterally, the ostomy presented an inclined and lateral aspect (Figs. 7.7 and 7.8), due to the septum pellucidum presenting in its lower limit with the floor of the frontal horn an inclination, following the form of the floor base and its relation with the head of the caudate nucleus (Fig. 7.8).
- Medially, the ostomy communicates with the left lateral ventricle through the septostomy. The ETSPR presented approximately 6 mm in diameter, corresponding approximately to the diameter of the endoscope trocar.

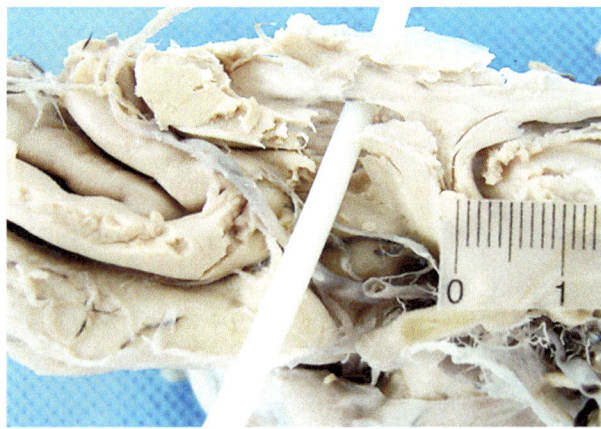

Fig. 7.6 Sagittal section of brain after ETSPR with a catheter through the ostomy. (Reprinted from Fuziki et al. [1]. With permission from Acta Cirurgica Brasileira)

Fig. 7.7 Superior view of an axial section of the brain at the level of the lateral ventricles showing the hole of the ETSPR. (Reprinted from Fuziki et al. [1]. With permission from Acta Cirurgica Brasileira)

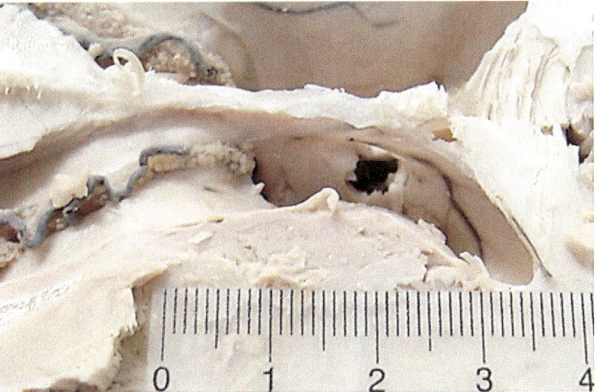

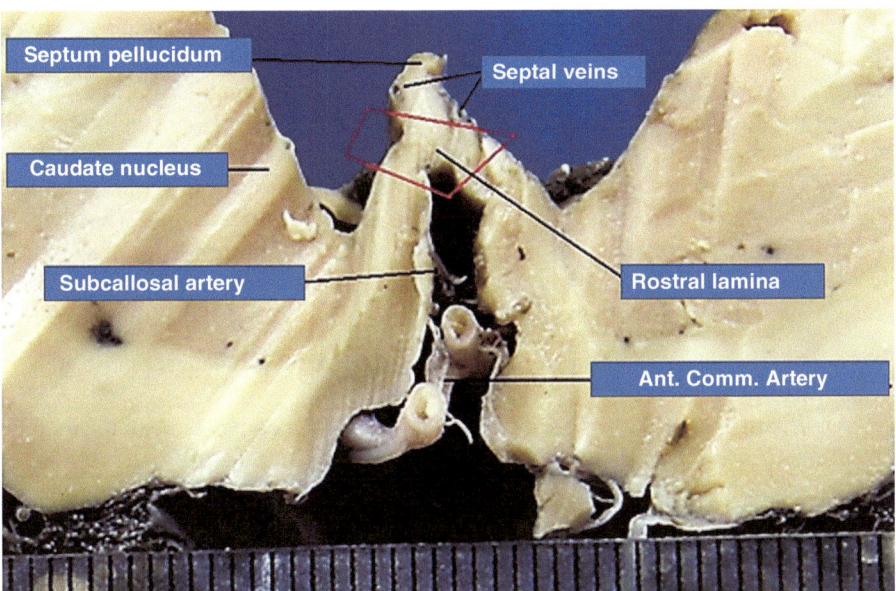

Fig. 7.8 Coronal section of the brain at the ostomy point, showing the anatomical relationship of the rostral lamina (lamina rostral) with the septum pellucidum and its inclined plane with the caudate nucleus on the frontal horn floor. The polygonal area in red is the site of the ETSPR. (Reprinted from Fuziki et al. [1]. With permission from Acta Cirurgica Brasileira)

7.4 Discussion

Contemporary surgical treatment of hydrocephalus consists of diversion of obstructed CSF transit through shunts to extracranial spaces, especially with ventriculoperitoneal shunts, and intracranial shunts through endoscopic fenestrations communicating the cerebral ventricles to cisterns of the subarachnoid space.

Although used for a long time, intracranial derivations remained in the ostracism until the improvement in technology with the development of endoscopy equipment that revitalized them [5–11]. The ETV, which consists of fenestration of the floor of the third ventricle, communicating it with the interpeduncular cistern, started to be used with great frequency in hydrocephalus due to obstruction of the cerebral ventricles [1–3]. However, in some situations ETV may become technically unviable, so the knowledge of internal derivations of the ventricular system alternatives becomes essential.

7.4.1   Floor of Frontal Horn and Hypothalamic-Septal Triangle

The rostrum of the corpus callosum in the sagittal section is gradually tapered in the posterior direction until it becomes a lamina, called the rostral lamina [12], whose posterior portion moves toward the fornix column, anterior commissure, and superior end of the lamina terminalis [13]. Superiorly, the rostral lamina is continuous with the leaflets of the pellucid septum and is located at the vertex of the intersection of the planes of the septum pellucidum with the floor of the frontal horn, thus forming a dihedral angle. The identification of the rostral lamina by direct superior view of the floor of the frontal horn or by endoscopic view of the ventricle is not possible because the septum pellucidum covers it, thus making its identification difficult. Below the rostral lamina is the hypothalamic-septal triangle [14] which has as limits (Fig. 7.1):

- A line joining the anterior face of the optic chiasm to the posterior portion of the anterior commissure
- A line connecting the posterior portion of the anterior commissure to the junction of the rostrum to the genu of the corpus callosum (commissuro-callosal line)
- A line joining the rostrum to the genu of the corpus callosum to the optic chiasm, closing the triangle

The structures contained in this triangle and its boundaries are the optic chiasm, the medial and lateral septal nuclei, the interstitial nuclei of the stria terminalis, the diagonal stria of the basilar part of the telencephalon (Broca's diagonal band), the accumbens nucleus, the nuclei of the anterior hypothalamus, the fibers of the anterior commissure, the fornix columns, the portions of the cingulus, the stria terminalis, the medullary striations of the thalamus, the medial fascicle of the telencephalon, and the fibers associated with the medial olfactory stria [13], as well as part of the A1 segments of the anterior cerebral arteries and the anterior communicating artery and its branches (hypothalamic, subcallosal, and median callosal arteries). The rostral lamina was identified in all anatomical specimens in the sagittal section. However, in the axial section, it is not visible because it is covered by the insertion of the septum pellucidum and its lower portion ends obliquely, bilaterally, in a small ramp toward the head of the caudate nucleus, with which it forms an angulation. Based on the proportion of means and the positive correlation between the interventricular foramen, the fornix column and the rostral lamina, as a reference point, a point anterior to the anterior edge of the interventricular foramen was determined, at a distance of approximately twice the diameter of this foramen, an ostomy was performed on two anatomical specimens in the rostral lamina (ETSPR), through which it was possible to reach the longitudinal fissure of the brain. The initial fenestration was performed with a 2 mm forceps at the base of the pellucid septum, directed at an acute angle, provided by the entrance of the endoscope through the cerebral cortex through the determined point, the same used in procedures such as the ETV. In the medial face of the frontal lobe, below the corpus callosum and before the anterior commissure, there is the paraolfactory area or subcallosal area [15, 16]. Its continuity in front of the lamina terminalis is the gyre or paraterminal body, also called the precommissural septum [15, 16]. The subcallosal gyrus and the paraterminal gyrus constitute the septal area, which is a component of the limbic system [12, 13, 15, 17–20]. The septal nuclei are located adjacent to the septum pellucidum. In animals, the septal nucleus presents medial and lateral components. In humans, the lateral septal nucleus may correspond to neurons located near the ventricular surface, while the medial septal nucleus corresponds to those near the septum pellucidum [20]. In addition, these medial cells are continuous with the gray substance on the medial surface of the cerebral hemispheres, in the rostral portion of the lamina terminalis. This region, called the paraterminal gyrus, joins with the core of the diagonal band of Broca, located at the base of the surface of the frontal pole [20]. Brodal reported the difficulty in identifying the septal nuclei in man and described that the upper part of the septal region forms the thin pellucid septum, which is devoid of nerve cells. The lower part of the precommissural septum is subdivided into a medial and lateral septal nucleus [15]. The medial (septum pellucidum), anterior (genu of the corpus callosum), and floor (rostrum of the corpus callosum) walls of the frontal horn of the lateral ventricle are drained by the anterior septal veins, which are formed by tributaries of the deep white matter near the frontal pole. They move medially through the floor and anterior wall to reach the septum pellucidum, are subsequently directed toward the interventricular foramen, contour the fornix above this foramen, enter the choroidal mesh, and end in the internal cerebral vein [21]. In the examination of the anatomical specimen under direct vision, the lateral limit of the ostomy presented a little distant from the midline due to the inclination of the floor of the lateral ventricle at the base of insertion of the septum pellucidum. The anterior limit of the ostomy reached a little beyond the rostral lamina reaching the rostrum of the corpus callosum, breaking some of its fibers, and its posterior limit was in front of the fornix column. Its medial portion of the ostomy performed by the right ventricle reached the left ventricle, passing under the septum pellucidum, and was identified through the visualization by the left lateral ventricle. Regarding the septal vein, the ostomy was located in an inferior position, before the junction of its tributaries. By the right ventricle ostomy, it was possible to identify just below, in the foreground, the subcallosal artery and, directing the endoscope in the anterior and inferior direction, the A2 segments of the left and right anterior cerebral arteries and the cortical portion of the left subcallosal area. Following with the endoscope in the lower and posterior directions, it was

Fig. 7.9 Subcallosal polygonal region (red lines) for access to subcallosal structures: anterior cerebral artery, anterior communicating artery, and optic chiasm, with its distances from rostral lamina (black lines). (Reprinted from Fuziki et al. [1]. With permission from Acta Cirurgica Brasileira)

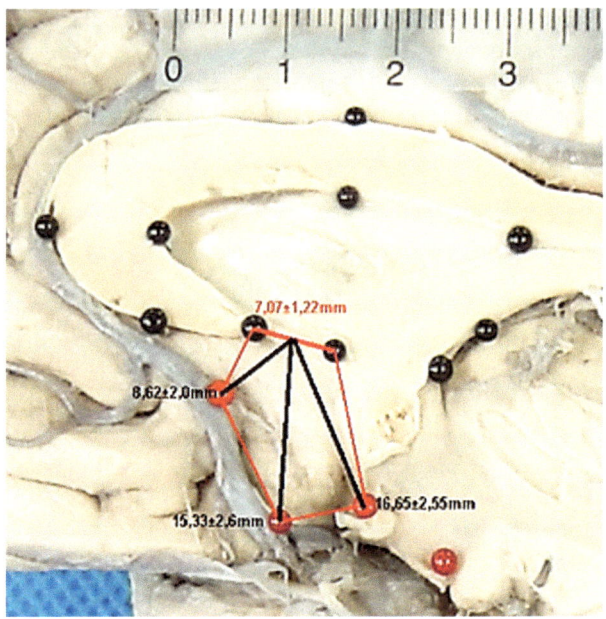

possible to visualize the optic chiasm, but this maneuver required the application of force in the endoscope against the cerebral parenchyma and against the posterior edge of the ostomy. During the inspection of the ostomy by the left ventricle, the left anterior cerebral artery and the right subcallosal area were visualized. The distances between the rostral lamina and the anterior cerebral arteries, the anterior communicating artery, and the supraoptic recess show the presence of a small polygonal area where it is possible to advance and work with the endoscope (Fig. 7.9).

7.4.2   Functional Considerations of Septal Area

Experiments in rats have shown that these animals prefer to receive electrical stimuli in the septal nucleus to receiving food and water and therefore it was judged to be the "area of pleasure," which would also play an important role in behaviors such as feeding and reproduction [20]. The septal syndrome, which occurs after the destruction of the septal nuclei in these animals, is described as an exacerbation of the behavioral reactions to the majority of environmental stimuli, which occur in the sexual and food spheres and in aggressive reactions [15]. Little is known about the function of the septal nucleus in humans. Observation in neurosurgical practice shows that the sectioning of the rostral lamina in surgeries for the treatment of calcified aneurysms and in ablative surgeries for the treatment of epilepsy, such as callosotomies and hemispherectomies, or accidental perforations of this lamina by ventricular catheters of derivations, are not accompanied by clinical manifestations attributable to specific lesions in this area.

7.4.3 Technical Feasibility of Endoscopic Fenestration

In this study it was demonstrated that endoscopic communication of the lateral ventricle with the longitudinal fissure of the brain through the ETSPR is anatomically possible. But would this communication present efficiency in the treatment of hydrocephalus? Would the CSF flow for the longitudinal fissure of the brain be sufficient to drain an obstructed ventricle, or would a larger cistern be necessary? Would the cerebrospinal fluid flow to the arachnoid villi in the cranial convexity allow its absorption? To analyze these questions, it is necessary to review two aspects of the CSF physiology, the first being where its absorption occurs and the second how its flow occurs. Cushing, in 1902, observed that there was a communication between the subarachnoid space and the sagittal sinus and that there would probably be a filter or valvular mechanism between the subarachnoid space and the venous sinuses [22, 23]. Since then, there is a wide acceptance that the communication for the passage of the cerebrospinal fluid is performed through the arachnoid villi. However, the exact nature of these channels and the mechanism of drainage of the CSF into the superior sagittal sinus are not fully understood [23–29]. More recently, other authors have demonstrated that the lymphatic system can play a considerable role in the process of CSF absorption, perhaps more important than that of arachnoid villi [30–35]. The action of arachnoid granulations as the main route for CSF is strongly questioned by Greitz and Hannerz [31], and the classic model of current flow of the CSF descending through the posterior region of the medulla and ascending through the anterior region was thus questioned for not clarifying the rapid distribution of the radionuclide and its large accumulation in the lumbar region. A pulsatile model for the CSF flow would better explain these facts and the accumulation of radionuclide in convexity, as well as its lightening in the region of the basal cisterns and in the cerebral parenchyma [31]. Critical to the absorption functions of arachnoid granulations are configured as the development of granulations does not occur until the closure of the fontanelle in children, no valvular mechanism was demonstrated in the granulations, marked albumin present in venous blood soon after its injection in the lumbar CSF, before being detected in the convexity region, and late presence of radioisotope in the convexity and in the lumbosacral region, indicating areas with reduced CSF exchange [32]. Greitz states that the CSF is absorbed by the cerebral capillaries and is transported through the subarachnoid spaces by vascular pulsation [32]. Based on the fact that cerebrospinal fluid production occurs throughout the nervous system, especially through the choroid plexus, and its absorption occurs through the cerebral capillaries, a hydrodynamic theory was proposed for the transport and absorption of CSF and its participation in the formation of hydrocephalus. In this model, arterial pulsations play an important role in the process of CSF flow, which occurs in a pulsatile way and not as a current flow, from the moment the CSF leaves the ventricular system and runs through the subarachnoid spaces until the moment it is absorbed by the cerebral capillaries [32]. The role of arterial pulse in the CSF flow is related to the compliance of the CSF compartment and the determination of intracranial pressure. This model is based on three premises: (1) in physiological conditions, the arterial pulse is converted into non-pulsatile venous flow by the action of arterial compliance, (2) the dynamic movement of the CSF through the foramen magnum is the primary facilitator of the occurrence of intracranial arterial expansion, and (3) the hydrostatic tissue pressure depends on the capillary hydrostatic pressure and the oncotic/osmotic pressure gradient created by the hemato-encephalic barrier [36]. In physiological conditions, based on the Monro-Kellie doctrine, the arterial systolic expansion drives the CSF through the foramen magnum and the venous blood to the venous sinuses, compressing the veins and bridges and producing venous flow. Venous compression increases retrograde pressure by dilating the venous capillaries during the cardiac cycle. At the same time, the arterial pulse wave dilates the arterial side of the capillaries by the *windkessel* effect (elastic capacity of the artery to release in the diastolic phase the arterial expansion absorbed in the systolic phase) and transforms the pulsating arterial flow into continuous capillary flow. Arterial expansion is essential for the *windkessel* effect and depends on intracranial compliance, which is directly related to dural sac compliance and compression of bridge veins [32]. Reducing compliance increases CSF pressure, but not enough to increase the difference in pressure to blood required for CSF absorption. The difference in pressure associated with reduced cerebral blood flow and increased capillary vascular resistance would be the factors responsible for CSF malabsorption [32]. The clinical improvement of patients submitted to treatments such as third ventriculostomy or insertion of a ventriculoperitoneal shunt in forms of hydrocephalus with restriction of intracranial compliance would occur not only by increasing the absorption of CSF but also by increasing intracranial compliance. A third ventriculostomy would increase ventricular outflow systolic flow, reduce intraventricular pulse pressure, and decrease ventricular width. This would dilate the compressed vessels and increase intracranial compliance, and the dilated capillaries would facilitate increased blood flow and CSF absorption. Similarly, the derivation would restore venous compliance because the CSF deviation causes a forced dilation of the compressed capacitor vessels [32]. Thus, a ventricular communication with the interhemispheric fissure by ETSPR could also increase intracranial compliance similar to the ETV, allowing the output of the CSF of the lateral ventricles, by its compression resulting from the expansion of the cerebral parenchyma and go through the subarachnoid spaces by means of transport by pulsating flow followed by subsequent absorption through the cerebral capillaries.

7.5 Conclusions

The rostral lamina is a constant structure in the human cerebral hemisphere and can be used as a site for fenestration, to communicate the lateral ventricle with the longitudinal fissure of the brain. The rostral lamina can be located under endoscopic view anterior to the fornix column using as reference the point before the limit of the interventricular foramen with the fornix column, at a distance equal to twice the anterior-posterior diameter of the interventricular foramen, at the limit between the inferior portion of the septum pellucidum and the floor of the frontal horn. The study of the main anatomical references related to the rostral lamina and the longitudinal fissure of the brain demonstrated that the perforation of the rostral lamina at the described site is safe, since there is a subcallosal polygonal cistern in the longitudinal fissure of the brain practically devoid of important anatomical structures, especially vascular ones.

References

1. Fuziki EJT, Dezena RA, Colli BO. Transseptumpellucidumrostrostomy: anatomical considerations and neuroendoscopic approach. Acta Cir Bras. 2011;26(Suppl 2):133–40. https://doi.org/10.1590/S0102-86502011000800025.
2. Gieger M, Cohen AR. The history of neuroendoscopy. In: Cohen AR, Hains SJ, editors. Minimally invasive technique in neurosurgery: concepts in neurosurgery. Baltimore: MD Williams & Wilkins; 1995. p. 1–5.
3. Li KW, Nelson C, Suk I, Jallo GI. Neuroendoscopy: past, present and future. Neurosurg Focus. 2005;19(6):E1.
4. Abbot R. History of neuroendoscopy. Neurosurg Clin N Am. 2004;15:1–7.
5. Andaluz N, Zucarello M. Fenestration of the lamina terminalis as a valuable adjunct in aneurysms surgery. Neurosurgery. 2004;55(5):1050–9.
6. Komotar RJ, Olivi A, Rigamonti D, Tamargo RJ. Microsurgical fenestration of the lamina terminalis reduces the incidence of shunt-dependent hydrocephalus after aneurismal subarachnoid hemorrhage. Neurosurgery. 2002;51(6):1403–12.
7. Kraemer JL, Gobbato PL, Andrade-Souza YM. Third ventriculostomy through the lamina terminalis for intracranial pressure monitoring after aneurysm surgery. Arq Neuropsiquiatr. 2002;60(4):932–4.
8. Sindou M. Favourable influence of opening the lamina terminalis and Lilliequist's membrane on the outcome of ruptured intracranial aneurysms: a study of 197 consecutive cases. Acta Neurochir. 1994;127:15–6.
9. Tomasello F, D'Avella D, de Divitiis O. Does lamina terminalis fenestration reduce the incidence of chronic hydrocephalus after subarachnoid hemorrhage. Neurosurgery. 1999;45(4):827.
10. Nakao N, Itakura T. Endoscopic lamina terminalis fenestration for treatment of hydrocephalus due to tuberculous meningitis. J Neurosurg. 2003;99:187.
11. Daniel RT, Lee GYF, Reilley PL. Suprapineal recess: an alternative site for third ventriculostomy? J Neurosurg. 2004;101:518–20.
12. Machado A. Neuroanatomia Funcional. São Paulo: A Atheneu; 1988.
13. Latarjet M, Liard AR. Anatomia humana. 2th ed. São Paulo: Panamericana; 1989.
14. Lancon JA, Haines DE, Raila FA, Parent AD, Vedanarayanan VV. Expanding cyst of the septum pellucidum. J Neurosurg. 1996;85:1127–34.
15. Brodal A. Anatomia Neurológica: com correlações clínicas. 3th ed. São Paulo: Editora Roca; 1979.
16. Comissão de Terminologia Anatômica. Sociedade Brasileira de Anatomia. Terminologia Anatômica Internacional. São Paulo: Editora Manole; 2001.
17. Citow JS, Macdonald RL. Neuroanatomia e Neurofisiologia: uma revisão. São Paulo: Livraria Santos Editora; 2004.
18. Gray H, Goss CM. Anatomia. 29.ed. Rio de Janeiro: Guanabara Koogan; 1988.
19. Kiernam JA. Neuroanatomia Humana de Barr. Barueri: Editora Manole; 2003.
20. Martin JH. Neuroanatomy: text and atlas. 2th ed. Stamford: Appleton & Lange; 1996.

21. Türe U, Yasargil GM, Krisht AF. The arteries of the corpus callosum: a microsurgical anatomic study. Neurosurgery. 1996;39(6):1075–85.
22. Jayatilaka ADP. An electron microscopic study of sheep arachnoid granulations. J Anat. 1965;99(3):635–49.
23. Yamashima T. Functional ultrastructure of cerebrospinal fluid drainage channels in human arachnoid villi. Neurosurgery. 1998;22(4):633–41.
24. Bergsneider M, Egnor MR, Johnston M, Kranz D, Madsen JR, Mcallister Ii JP, et al. What we don't (but should) know about hydrocephalus. J Neurosurg. 2006;104(3 Suppl Pediatrics):157–9.
25. Conegero CI, Chopard RP. Tridimensional architecture of the collagen element in the arachnoid granulations in humans. Arq Neuropsiquiatr. 2003;61(3-A):561–5.
26. Davson H, Domer FR, Hollingsworth JR. The mechanism of drainage of cerebrospinal fluid. Brain. 1973;96:329–36.
27. Fox RJ, Walji AH, Mielke B, Petruk KC, Aronyk KE. Anatomic details of intradural channels in the parasagittal dura: a possible pathway for flow of cerebrospinal fluid. Neurosurgery. 1996;39(1):84–91.
28. Go GK, Houthoff H, Hartsuiker J, Blaauw EH, Havinga P. Fluid secretion in arachnoid cysts as a clue to cerebrospinal fluid absorption at arachnoid granulation. J Neurosurg. 1986;65:642–8.
29. Mawera G, Asala SA. The function of arachnoid villi/granulations revisited. Central Afr J Med. 1996;42(9):281–4.
30. Boulton M, Armstrong D, Flessner M, Hay J, Szalai JP, Johnston M. Raised intracranial pressure increases CSF drainage through arachnoid villi and extracranial lymphatics. Am J Physiol Regul Integr Comp Physiol. 1998;275(44):889–96.
31. Greitz D, Hannerz J. A proposed model of cerebrospinal fluid circulation: observations with radionuclide cisternography. Am J Neuroradiol. 1996;17:431–8.
32. Greitz D. Radiological assessment of hydrocephalus: new theories and implications for therapy. Neurosurg Rev. 2004;27:145–65.
33. Johnston M, Zakharov A, Koh L, Armstrong D. Subarachnoid injection of microfil reveals connections between cerebrospinal fluid and nasal lymphatics in trh non-human primate. Neuropathol Appl Neurobiol. 2005;31(6):632.
34. Mollanji R, Bozanovic-Sosic R, Zakharov A, Makarian L, Johnston MG. Blocking cerebrospinal fluid absorption through the cribriform plate increases resting intracranial pressure. Am J Physiol Regul Integr Comp Physiol. 2002;282:1593–9.
35. Papaiconomou C, Bozanovic-Sosic R, Zakharov A, Johnston M. Does neonatal cerebrospinal fluid absorption occur via arachnoid projections or extracranial lymphatics? Am J Physiol Regul Integr Comp Physiol. 2002;283:869–76.
36. Bergsneider M, Alwan AA, Falkson L, Rubinstein EH. The relationship of pulsatile cerebrospinal fluid flow to cerebral flow and intracranial pressure: a new theoretical model. Acta Neurochir. 1998;71(Suppl):266–8.

Index

© Springer Nature Switzerland AG 2020
R. A. Dezena, *Endoscopic Third Ventriculostomy*,
https://doi.org/10.1007/978-3-030-28657-6